GOING LEAN

Busting Barriers to Patient Flow

GOING LEAN

Busting Barriers to Patient Flow

Amy C. Smith

Robert Barry

Clifford E. Brubaker

HAP

ACHE Management Series

Your board, staff, or clients may also benefit from this book's insight. For more information on quantity discounts, contact the Health Administration Press Marketing Manager at (312) 424-9470.

12 11 10 09 08   5 4 3 2 1

Library of Congress Cataloging-in-Publication Data

Smith, Amy C., 1964-
 Going lean : busting barriers to patient flow / Amy C. Smith, Robert Barry, and Clifford E. Brubaker.
    p. ; cm.
  ISBN-13: 978-1-56793-281-2 (alk. paper)
1. Health facilities--Administration. 2. Hospital care--Quality control. 3. Total quality management. 4. Patient satisfaction. 5. Hospital utilization. I. Barry, Robert, 1938 Dec. 29- II. Brubaker, Cliff. III. Title. [DNLM: 1. Health Facilities--organization & administration. 2. Hospital Administration--methods. 3. Hospital-Patient Relations. 4. Hospitalization. 5. Quality Control. 6. Total Quality Management. WX 153 S642g 2007]
  RA971.S616 2007
  362.1068--dc22

                                                    2007035574

The paper used in this publication meets the minimum requirements of American National Standard for Information Sciences—Permanence of Paper for Printed Library Materials, ANSI Z39.48-1984. ⊗™

Acquisitions editor: Audrey Kaufman; Project manager: Jane Calayag; Cover designer and layout editor: Chris Underdown

Health Administration Press
A division of the Foundation of the
   American College of Healthcare Executives
1 North Franklin Street, Suite 1700
Chicago, IL 60606-3529
(312) 424-2800

Contents

Foreword

Why is this patient still here?

The answers to that question, according to the authors of this well-documented, clearly written book, are crucial determinants of healthcare quality and efficiency. The authors, several of whom are certified as Six Sigma Black Belts or Master Black Belts, deftly integrate theory and practice while providing numerous examples of initiatives that are improving patient care and system economies with the use of Lean principles. *Going Lean: Busting Barriers to Patient Flow* is an excellent sequel to the authors' previous, acclaimed contribution to quality care, *The Six Sigma Book for Healthcare: Improving Outcomes by Reducing Errors.*

This informative, readable work reflects the evolution and refinement of the authors' thinking on this topic. It is also a collection of the productive results achieved by a wide variety of healthcare organizations that have applied the Lean principles. In the Lean perspective, the correct measure of healthcare quality and efficiency is patient flow. In the authors' view, the highest priority of all systems and subsystems should be discharging patients to the home or to another level of care as quickly and as medically appropriate as possible. Length of stay should be measured, the authors correctly argue, *in hours, not days!*

Although Lean principles can be easily understood and readily applied in healthcare environments, they require an organization to shift the focus and priorities of its systems and subsystems. Designed to achieve exactly the results they are producing, these existing systems are based on efficiencies relative to their internal priorities. For example, clinical laboratories often batch tests for production efficiency. But in organizations that are focused on patient flow, the greater priority is to expedite the lab test so that care providers can have rapid access to the results and so that treatment or therapy can be quickly implemented or modified, thus improving patient flow. Some costs, the authors assert, may have to be suboptimized to achieve optimal patient flow.

All of the examples presented in this book, some of which could be regarded as breakthrough strategies, show measurable, sustainable improvements. Among the various changes in structures and processes, those that generally enjoyed the greatest success were the ones openly sponsored or endorsed by top management. This helped dissipate upstream or downstream institutional barriers.

This book, which is a superior reference for healthcare governance, leaders, managers, and clinicians, offers abundant insights into and recommendations for simultaneously maximizing patient care quality and operations efficiency. Among these suggestions are (1) assigning hospitalists as attending physicians to help improve patient flow and (2) clearly displaying measured improvements and progress reports on charts or dashboards to maintain organizational focus. As is often emphasized in business schools, what gets measured and reported usually gets accomplished.

Other important recommendations in the book include the following:

- Senior managers should spend more time observing care processes and monitoring targeted outcomes.
- Compensation practices, especially incentive compensation, should favor the improvement of patient flow.
- Senior management should encourage standardization where possible.

- Organizations should sponsor a small number of breakthrough projects that are highly visible, and senior management should openly sponsor the change process.
- Healthcare organizations should establish an admission and discharge control desk to enhance patient flow and optimal use of inpatient resources.
- Healthcare organizations should establish distinct observation units and licensed buffer care facilities.

The U.S. healthcare system needs to address major quality issues, on both macro and micro levels. Applying the principles of evidence-based medicine, external benchmarking, and redesigning patient care processes hold great promise that will help healthcare leaders resolve significant quality concerns. In healthcare, we expend a large and growing percentage of the gross domestic product, but we don't necessarily produce benefits for the overall health status of our population. We have major problems with the uninsured, and healthcare costs are affecting our ability to compete in the global economy.

We can and must do better! Thankfully, *Going Lean* can help us do that. It provides exceptional guidance for accomplishing urgently demanded improvements in healthcare quality and efficiency. I encourage you to read this book. You'll be glad you did. And remember to ask, Why is this patient still here?

Ronald R. Aldrich, FACHE,
healthcare governance consultant,
Limberpine Associates, Inc.,
Dubois, Wyoming

Preface

Why is this patient still here?

That's the patient-flow issue in a nut shell. In senior-management terms, with every department working at maximum efficiency and high productivity, why is this patient still here?

Why? Because maximum efficiency for each department and maximum efficiency for all departments taken together are not the same as minimizing the time to complete treatment of the patient. Therefore, the patient is still here. Moreover, being efficient goes in the wrong direction. Isn't that maddening? Overcoming the urge to be efficient takes some doing. Lots of people have done it, though, and our book is replete with success stories. Let's illustrate the difference between efficiency and time minimization with the following example.

Suppose you walk into a medical arts office building and go to the lobby to find an elevator that goes up to the fourth floor. Suppose there is only one elevator—a big one—and you get to it just as the elevator doors are about to close. You jump in, smile to one and all, and make a quick trip up to the fourth floor.

Suppose, instead, that you just missed the closing doors and now have to wait patiently, or impatiently, until the elevator car goes up and comes back down again. While you're waiting, other folks will have joined you. The elevator eventually comes back down, then in and up you all go. That's efficient. For the elevator. Full load almost every time. Passengers conform to what the elevator wants to do.

Now suppose that the building had been built with two half-size elevators. The service rendered to the passenger is exactly the same, and the waiting time for the least-lucky passenger would be cut in half. But now, the efficiency is down because two half-size elevators cost more than one full-size elevator, two take up more building space, and one will run with a light load most of the day. Less efficient. For the elevators.

It would be nice to have individual elevator cars for each passenger, like a taxi service. Minimum waiting, but very poor elevator efficiency. Escalators, which are expensive and slow compared to an elevator, give each passenger an individual "car" in the form of a step to stand on. Minimum waiting, but low efficiency.

This example addresses only one activity. If you have to wait for a bus, change buses, wait in queue to get through the building's revolving door, and then take the elevator, this efficiency question comes up again and again and again. Stage by stage, efficiency is simply not the same thing as minimum time to complete the process.

Certainly there are constraints. The building is only so big and cannot be given over entirely to elevator shafts. Once the building is built, it's really hard to add an elevator to cope with increased demand. You, the passenger, are left to cope with completely different providers along the way, and those providers have every reason to maximize their own efficiency and share only a vague interest in the totality of the service provided to you.

A healthcare patient may see the same multiplicity of independent providers as seen by an elevator passenger. But, in healthcare, often enough there are a series of steps under the nominal control of a common entity, perhaps a hospital. That common entity, at the senior level, has some freedom to choose efficiency on the one hand or patient flow on the other. Patient flow and minimum total treatment time are related. Maximum patient flow goes with maximum revenue as well as maximum consideration of the patient's time. But if the system is geared for maximum efficiency, can it be re-geared for maximum patient flow?

That's what this book is about, with lots of success stories.

We propose to you the Lean Method as a straightforward, systematic management approach to improving patient flow, maximizing the beneficial utilization of key resources, and getting to the point where you will know the answer (and it will be a good one) to "why is this patient still here?"

Senior management, having decided to change direction, will necessarily be working through others to effect the change in direction. This book offers help in that regard, helping the reader to characterize the reader's present system, explain to others what's desired, and measure progress along the way. No statistics, just simple tracking of the patient's progress through the system.

The other task left to senior management is to figure out how the present system rewards present performance (efficiency) and how the reward system needs to be altered to reward a different sort of performance (patient flow). Exhortation isn't enough. The reward system needs attention.

This book also talks about organization. Healthcare systems have lots of people who are keenly interested in healthcare tasks. Not many have a longitudinal interest in keeping the patient moving along. Case managers do, service line managers might, but not many others beyond that. Certainly most caregivers need to retain that task focus, and yet the longitudinal interest needs to be there.

In this book, we are pleased to have contributions from practitioners who are telling their own success stories. Mr. Mark Hernandez helped us with the Army Medical Command's success story in Chapter 5. Ms. Becky Southern and Mr. Mark Viau contributed mightily to the telling of their Boca Raton Women's Center success story in Chapter 8. An abbreviated bio for each of our special contributors is included in the About the Contributors section at the end of the book.

We take this opportunity to salute the leadership of Colonel (Ret.) Gaston M. "Randy" Randolph, Jr., who has recently retired from active military service. Now a civilian, he has taken up new challenges as director of Enterprise Innovation for the U.S. Army Medical Command (MEDCOM), Office of the Surgeon General. Randy directs Lean, Six Sigma, balanced scorecard, and other MEDCOM improvement initiatives worldwide.

Finally, we wish to express our gratitude to and admiration for the following institutions and departments who granted us the privilege of including their success stories in this book and whose management took the time and trouble to add to and correct our telling of their stories. Any abiding errata are our doing, not theirs.

- Army Medical Command
- Boca Raton Community Hospital
- Conemaugh Health System
- Heritage Valley Health System
- Highmark, Inc.
- Pennsylvania Health Care Cost Containment Council
- Pittsburgh Regional Health Initiative
- University of Pittsburgh Medical Center (UPMC) information technology
- UPMC Shadyside Hospital pathology laboratory
- UPMC Winter Institute for Simulation, Education, and Research
- Veterans Administration Pittsburgh Healthcare System
- Virginia Mason Medical Center
- Western Pennsylvania Hospital—Forbes Regional Campus (part of West Penn Allegheny Health System)
- Western Reserve Care System

PART I

GETTING STARTED

We introduce the Lean Method for healthcare. We encourage you to think in terms of barriers and bottlenecks. We explain how Lean deals with barriers and bottlenecks to improve patient flow.

CHAPTER 1

Introduction

The Lean Management Method moves healthcare from its traditional task orientation to patient-flow orientation to provide better patient service, better patient care, and better utilization of assets.

Everybody is in favor of better patient flow. Patients, providers, payers—everybody is in favor of moving the patient more briskly and smoothly through the system.

Better patient flow is possible. In this book, we have included a nice sampling of success stories, both to celebrate the trailblazers and to show our readers that it really can be done.

> Your system is perfectly designed to produce the results you are now getting.
>
> —Attributed to W. E. Deming

This book is about the Lean Method, which is easy to understand, easy to visualize, and easy to apply.

We'll get to Lean shortly. First, let's spend a few minutes on the senior executive's issues with managing change, because instituting Lean is a change. Nobel Laureate Herbert Simon taught that the hardest things for the senior manager who wishes to make changes to get different (better, one supposes) results are these (Raden 2007):

1. how to get the important problems to the top of the management agenda,
2. how to represent the issues in a way that others can understand them, and
3. how to represent the issues in a way that facilitates solutions.

Professor Simon came to the conclusion that once these things were in hand, interested parties could proceed to find solutions. Bright people are pretty good at solving well-defined problems. Healthcare is replete with bright people.

Patient flow as a topic is already pretty near the top of every healthcare executive's agenda, so the first question posed by Professor Simon is satisfied to start with, and we're off to a good start. Lean helps with the other two, providing a representation that people understand readily and providing a structure that encourages everybody, each in his own interest, to move the system in the right direction.

Where are we now? Healthcare systems are professionally managed and highly optimized today. Changing the system must, therefore, move the system away from its present optimized state. Can that be a good idea? Yes, because the present system is composed of a number of stages of production, each of which is optimized to be the most efficient it can possibly be, on its own. That's not the same as being optimized overall, and it's not the same thing as being optimized for best patient flow. Optimizing for best patient flow moves some stages of production away from local optima and increased local cost. The benefit comes in higher throughput, moving patients through the entire system, end to end, more quickly. That's the fundamental idea of Lean. It's not at all a matter of working harder or even working smarter. It's a matter of applying different measures of success.

Lean provides not only a systematic way to define success—improved patient flow—Lean also provides the visualization necessary to teach others about the present system and how it can be improved. This responds to Professor Simon's second question.

Finally, Lean provides a systematic way to encourage middle managers to move the system in the right direction. Healthcare has a famously weak authority structure, so it is necessary to find ways so that all the independent actors want to go in the preferred direction for their own reasons.

It can be done. Real hospitals, real clinics, real laboratories with real patients have shown it can be done. Success stories are included in this book. Imitating the successful is a pretty good way to make progress. Your people are just as bright and just as keen on improving healthcare as those who appear in our success stories. Maybe more so.

This book is written for senior managers, present and future. Senior managers determine policy and direction, creating rewards systems to motivate people to go in the desired direction. Senior managers allocate capital and authorize budgets. Junior managers execute the policy, apply the capital, and operate within budgets. There are some things junior managers, no matter how bright and energetic, simply can't do. Some participation by both senior and junior management will be required.

It's not likely that big reorganizations will be required to benefit from Lean. Today, hospitals commonly have service line managers and case managers, both of whom can be powerful forces in improving patient flow. Today, many hospitals have hospitalists—physicians whose full-time occupation is to act as attending physicians. A good part of improving patient flow relies on the cooperation of physicians, and it is easier to deal with a small number of hospitalists than with a huge number of admitting physicians. Indeed, Medicare changes for 2007, which go even further in the direction of paying hospitals on the basis of what physicians write in the patient's record, make hospitalists all the more attractive to any hospital.

Healthcare is, even today, a matter of people dealing with people. Most of the issues in the field are people issues, and nothing can be done in healthcare without the cooperation of lots of people holding varying interests and perceptions. Even with all of today's machines and computers, people make the system go. Or not go.

Each patient is precious. Each improvement in the system's operations must surely go in the direction of improving patient care. Optimizing must be done in the patient's favor. Happily, doing this improves patient flow.

This book is jargon free—no Latin, no Greek. Very few acronyms, other than CEO (chief executive officer).

THAT'S THE GOVERNOR ON THAT STRETCHER!

The ambulance arrives. The trauma team is ready. Blood samples are drawn and sent by courier to the lab, where technicians are standing by. The trauma team's leader orders an x-ray, so the patient is rolled directly to the x-ray department, where technicians and a radiologist are standing by.

Exploratory surgery is ordered; surgeons, anesthesiologists, and surgical nurses are standing by. A surgical theater is cleared and prepped. Post-op space is freed up, and the intensive care unit is standing by. Meanwhile, the admissions department is told to retrofit insurance formalities as the case unfolds. A skilled nursing home, a rehabilitation hospital, and a home nursing service are put on notice to stand by for later information and to be ready to accept the patient.

All utterances of the patient's attending physicians are transmitted in real time to the medical transcription service, to transcribe on the fly and to return for signature. The same goes for nurses' care plans and reports. Discharge orders are prepared in advance, including take-home instructions for medicine, therapy, and follow-up care. An ambulance is ordered to stand by for the earliest possible discharge of this precious patient.

Oops! It Isn't the Governor After All!

Okay, so it's not the governor. It's a regular citizen who would certainly benefit from and appreciate the same intensity of focus that the governor would get. More likely, today, the citizen-patient would find that, in nearly every department, providers are already busy taking care of previous patients as efficiently as they possibly can. Because the providers are already busy, our citizen-patient is going to have to wait a few minutes. Or more. At every step along the way.

What's the Difference?

The medical care given to the governor and to the citizen is the same. The difference is not in the care; it is in the time it takes, overall, to get that care. The no-delay mode works for the governor. Can it be made to work for the citizen, too?

Yes, by getting the queuing time to shrink to nearly nothing and by a proper understanding of each department's role in patient flow. Should the x-ray department have technicians standing around, just in case a patient shows up? Maybe. Should the lab have idle lab techs? Maybe. Doesn't that cost money? Yes. Doesn't that waste money? Maybe not.

Lean is here to help sort those things out. Lean provides a visualization mechanism, an understanding of the overall system, and a method for getting everybody's self-interest to promote better patient flow. Why better patient flow? More revenue for the same productive assets, happier patients, happier staff. Unity of focus.

Patient flow is good.

Reference

Raden, N. 2007. "Toppling the BI Pyramid." *DM Review* Magazine (January): 28.

CHAPTER 2

The Lean Method

Find nonproductive time in the patient's treatment, then clear it away.

Apply Lean to remove nonproductive time, as viewed by individual patients. A Lean process is optimized in this one regard—minimum time as counted by the patient. A Lean process may cost more, and it may take more effort. By providing better patient flow, a Lean process overcomes those negatives.

Minimizing patient time is the same as maximizing patient flow. Lean maximizes patient flow. Maximum patient flow means maximum utilization of key assets. Because key assets are finite, there is a physical limit on what the maximum patient flow can be.

If it were possible to expand the capacity of those key assets by simple means, then the logical thing to do would be to expand. However, key assets are almost always limited by regulation, by practical physical size, or by an outsized capital cost to get an increase in key capacity. That's the bottleneck. There is always one bottleneck in any real system, one productive element that just can't be expanded.

If there is one element that is the bottleneck, then there are other elements that are not bottlenecks. Not being bottlenecks, they can be expanded or redirected to improve patient flow. In real systems, the bottleneck is well known to senior management and is already getting a lot of attention. Big payoffs in patient flow improvement will likely come from figuring out why those nonbottleneck elements are detracting from patient flow and doing something about it. What barriers to patient flow exist in those non-bottleneck units? Can something be done?

Yes. Others have already done so. Lean provides a systematic way of identifying and dealing with barriers. Bottlenecks and barriers are keys to the Lean Method.

VISUALIZING PATIENT FLOW

Consider the flow of a typical treatment as portrayed in the simple flowchart in Figure 2.1. The essential characteristics are that there are some upstream steps, a bottleneck, and one or more downstream steps. The number of upstream and downstream steps may be many, but the number of bottlenecks is always only one. One process, one bottleneck.

Figure 2.1. Elementary Flowchart

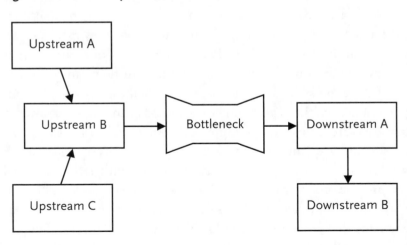

The flowchart is only half the story. We also need to visualize how value is being added, and over what time period, as the patient progresses through the system (see Figure 2.2). In plotting value-added versus time, anything that adds value to the patient's treatment moves the line up the page. When no value is being added, then the line does not move up the page, it just moves to the right as time goes by. The patient is waiting. Nothing is happening. No value is being added.

The value-added chart is notional. It doesn't make any difference what the scale is. What matters is that there are flat spots. When the governor was the patient, there were no flat spots. If you can do it for the governor, can you do it for everybody?

At the bottleneck point in the treatment, physical limits come into play. If there is only one MRI (magnetic resonance imaging) machine and five patients are waiting, then the next patient is going to have to wait. At nonbottleneck steps, though, it would not take big money or regulatory relief to expand production, so why is the patient made to wait? Almost always, the answer is that the nonbottleneck step is optimized to minimize cost. Local optimization

Figure 2.2. Value Added Versus Time Chart

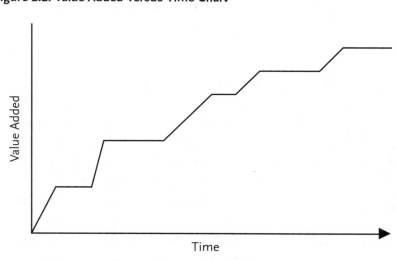

minimizes local cost. To get an improvement in patient flow, the local management needs to be persuaded to give up some benefit for the overall good of the patient.

Lean helps management identify the barriers. Dealing with them will still be up to senior management. For instance, if cardiologists don't want to work weekends doing nonemergency catheterizations (so patients admitted on Friday afternoon wait until Monday morning, with no value being added for two-plus days), that's a barrier. Can management do something about it? Yes. It might take a lot of negotiating, it might cost some money, but it can be done.

At the bottleneck, it is often useful to treat patients in a batch to maximize bottleneck throughput. Given that the bottleneck limits overall production, batching may be appropriate at the bottleneck. Batching is almost never appropriate at nonbottleneck points. Batching means that patients are kept in queue while the batch is formed, so batching means longer total treatment time. Batching at nonbottleneck points goes in the wrong direction.

Why is it done? To improve the local efficiency. De-batching, or working with smaller batches rather than large ones, goes in the right direction. The right batch size, away from the bottleneck, is one solution. One patient. Batch of one.

If batch of one can be made to work at the bottleneck too, so much the better.

BOTTLENECKS ARE GOOD, BARRIERS ARE BAD

A bottleneck is the part of the system that is so hard or so expensive to increase in size that it limits the capacity of the entire system.

Bottlenecks are good? Yes, because a bottleneck is a limitation on the ability of others to enter and compete for your business. Bottlenecks defend those already in the business and discourage and even block others from entering. Bottlenecks make it hard for a competitor to expand capacity and take business away. So, bottlenecks are good. Let's be clear about what we mean by the term "bottleneck."

A bottleneck is the part of the system that is so hard or so expensive to increase in size that it limits the capacity of the entire system.

What then is a "barrier?"

A barrier is a self-imposed limit on production. Why would anyone self-impose a limit on production? To meet objectives that were correct when they were set. Maybe they aren't the right objectives today. But when they were set, it was very likely that efficiency at each stage of care was considered to be the best overall strategy. To be efficient on its own, each stage organized its work to minimize the time and effort needed to do all the work assigned to it.

To be most efficient, get all the inputs together and do the work in one big batch, using the biggest tools and machines available. A pathology lab, for instance, would gather up all the tissue samples and process them in a batch. That's the most efficient way to get the *last* tissue sample done, but it's the least efficient way to get the *first* tissue sample done (because the first one just waits there until the last one is ready to start). With this most efficient lab strategy, the first patient waits an extra-long time to get a result. So does the average patient and every patient afterward, except the very last one in the batch. This policy is optimum for the pathology lab itself. It's a good policy if the objective of the system is to have the most efficient pathology lab. It's not the best policy if the overall objective of the system is to get lab results back as soon as possible for each patient so that treatment can proceed.

The pathology lab can, of course, work with single tissue samples or in small batches if ordered to do so, and it will continue to do so if appropriately encouraged, rewarded, and not punished— that is to say, when a coherent set of policies is applied to move from maximizing lab efficiency to maximizing patient flow. The lab, as a result, will be somewhat less efficient than before. The same applies to all units involved in the patient's care, many more than just the pathology lab. (For a pathology lab success story, see Chapter 11.)

In short, the barriers that inhibit patient flow today were put in place for sound reasons, but those reasons are no longer predominant.

ACCELERATING PATIENT FLOW

Through the Bottleneck

> There is one bottleneck, and that bottleneck limits production.

The patient flows through a series of steps or stages in the care process. Exactly one of those stages is the bottleneck. The others are not bottlenecks. There are never two bottlenecks in any process.

In addition to the bottleneck, there are one or more stages upstream and one or more stages downstream. All upstream stages feed into the bottleneck, and all downstream stages flow away from the bottleneck. There are never bypasses around the bottleneck, because if there were, it wouldn't be a bottleneck!

There can be lots of other obstructions in the system, but there is only one bottleneck. Why only one? Because it always works out that way.

Let's take an MRI center, because it is easy to visualize. The bottleneck is the expensive MRI machine. Suppose the admissions office is sized to match exactly the number of patients the MRI machine can process in a day. Would that mean there are two bottlenecks? No, because the admissions office can be expanded with little money, comparatively speaking, to have a larger capacity than the MRI machine itself; therefore, the admissions office does not qualify as a bottleneck. That is to say, if management had some reason to expand the admissions office, then the admissions office would be expanded.

> Some MRI centers in Canada, which are few in number and have long patient queues, do not scan patients on the night shift; they scan pets to create a cash business (Frogue et al. 2001). Finding a new market is a tried-and-true way of dealing with excess capacity.

On the other hand, if management wanted to expand the MRI machine capacity, management would have to find some serious money to put on the table before doing so. The management action required is of a different magnitude.

The bottleneck limits the capacity of the system. No matter what is done elsewhere in the system, no "product" goes through the system without going through the bottleneck. Time lost in the bottleneck is lost forever and cannot be recovered. Therefore, any lost time in the bottleneck is a big deal. All upsets in the bottleneck—including supply outages, equipment outages, operating errors, patient no-shows, unauthorized work, and lost records—need to be anticipated and thwarted beforehand. Time gained at the bottleneck improves patient flow. Time gained at the bottleneck improves the true capacity of the entire system because more patients can be treated in the same total time.

In rebuttal, it may be said, "We can always work an extra shift to catch up." If you have an unworked shift, then you have idle bottleneck capacity. Why is that? Expensive capacity not being used, on purpose? Is business being turned away? It may be said, "We don't have enough demand to stay busy all the time. We can use the slack to catch up." If so, then capacity ought to be reduced, freeing up assets and staff for more productive purposes than this nonproduction. It may be said, "We can catch up by working a little faster for an hour or so." Would corners be cut? Why not work faster all the time, then?

It may be said, "We can catch up by moving some of the work out of the bottleneck and over to another point in the system." Fine, do it that way all the time. It may be said, "We can catch up by doing extra work ahead of time so that the bottleneck time is reduced. Oh, but we'd have to hire three more technicians to do the extra non-bottleneck work, and our expenses would go up in that other department." Revenue increase will surely repay the added expense very quickly.

The bottleneck may be an expensive machine, the bottleneck may be the limited availability of surgical nurses, or the bottleneck may be a regulatory limit on the number of beds. Whatever the bottleneck is, it's something that is hard to expand. Managers at the bottleneck see that their own performance is measured first of all by production through the bottleneck. Conflicting goals are unlikely to arise. That's good; it makes things easy for senior management.

At the bottleneck, the local optimum always supports good patient flow.

At the bottleneck, there are many potential barriers to production, hence to patient flow, and we will deal with those later in the chapter. First, let's identify and give names to the nonbottleneck elements in the system.

Through Upstream Stages

It is easy to see that upsets located upstream of the bottleneck may starve the bottleneck of work to be done. Consider that MRI center again. If no patients are waiting, if the waiting patients are not qualified for one reason or another, or if the waiting patients are not coached on what to expect and thus balk, then the bottleneck will be idle and revenue will be lost forever. It is tempting to order patients to arrive hours before their time slot just to make sure that at least one patient is waiting to go in. But patient flow is counted on the patient's clock, and extra-early-arrival scheduling scores badly and drives business away.

> The sole purpose of the stage(s) of production upstream of the bottleneck is to keep the bottleneck busy generating revenue.

Well, if extra-early arrival is ruled out, what's left? Dealing with the barriers to orderly and timely patient flow. We will come back to barrier clearing later.

Having a patient ready when the bottleneck is ready—that's the only point. That's what the upstream stages are supposed to do. If no patient is ready when the bottleneck is ready, bottleneck capacity goes unused, revenue falls, and smiles fade.

Should more that one patient be poised in readiness? That depends on the variability of the upstream stages. If patients sometimes don't show up or are tardy, if identification is lacking, if payer formalities are not cleared, or if there are physical obstructions, then the upstream stage can be highly variable. Handling several patients upstream at the same time invites variability because it invites confusion. So the temptation is to bring in patients well ahead of time and let them wait, just to cover the variability and to make sure a patient is ready when the bottleneck is ready. That goes against good patient flow, as experienced by the patient doing the waiting.

Dealing with variability starts with sorting out what variability is controllable and what variability is not. Control the controllable variability with careful process design and execution; hedge against the uncontrollable variability. We'll get back to this, after we introduce the downstream stages.

Through Downstream Stages

Patient flow downstream is maximized by minimizing the time each patient is present at this stage. The appropriate measure of patient flow starts with the patient's view of the process. Shortening the downstream time is good.

Completing the work downstream in a satisfactory way includes reducing, to the greatest extent possible, any likelihood that the bottleneck treatment will have to be repeated on the patient. After all, if the patient has to make another trip through the bottleneck, then that patient is taking up space that another patient would otherwise have filled. Suppose an upset occurs downstream, and everything stops there for a period of time. That's an inconvenience for the patients affected, but it does not reduce overall production. Downstream has excess capacity, compared to the bottleneck, so this stage will catch up. Downstream has slack, so there is no reason to cut any corners to catch up. Idle time downstream will go down for the period of time necessary to catch up, and that's okay.

Downstream with no upsets has idle time. That's good. Management must resist the temptation to reduce downstream capacity, which creates a barrier. Downstream with no upsets needs to have some idle time, some excess capacity, so that catching up can happen if an upset occurs. Downstream with no upsets can soak up some of its idle time by giving each patient individual attention. It might be more efficient to gather patients together in batches for downstream

> The sole purpose of the stage(s) of production downstream of the bottleneck is to complete the work.

processing, but that is to the disadvantage of the patient. Individual attention downstream is the best policy. The patients will love it.

Doing things—like handling two patients at a time—to reduce local effort minutes is optimizing locally, optimizing in a way to please the productive unit at the inconvenience of the patient while slowing down the overall process.

Optimizing in favor of the patient is always the same as optimizing in favor of the system as a whole. Local optimization is to be discouraged. Improving the downstream process to reduce the processing time for individual patients is still worthwhile, because that improves overall cycle time as counted by the patient.

Push and Pull

Push and pull are meaningful and terse words to describe the best ways to operate at each stage.

Upstream is *pull*. When the bottleneck is ready for the next patient, a patient is pulled to the bottleneck from the upstream stage. The upstream stage then bestirs itself to get another patient ready. The control rests with the bottleneck; the upstream stage just responds to the pull order.

The bottleneck itself is *push*. Each patient is pushed through the bottleneck treatment process with the minimum of lost time. Downstream is *push*. Each patient's treatment is completed as briskly as possible.

All stages work with the smallest practicable batches of patients, blood samples, tissue samples, and so on. The goal is to operate on a batch-of-one production basis because that gives the fastest completion of the patient's treatment.

GETTING LEAN, STEP BY STEP

Experience shows that good results flow from following the steps given here.

- *Observe.* Go watch patients in the waiting room. Follow a few all the way through the process. Sketch some value-added versus time charts. Find out what peer organizations and other industries are doing.
- *Set the goal.* The *goal* is what an ideal system would produce. Keep the goal in mind so that all the changes you introduce go in the right direction.

A *specification* is a quantitative pass/fail test of performance. So, while the goal is to answer every telephone call before the first ring; the specification might be to answer 95 percent of busy-hour calls before the fourth ring. Meeting the specification is the minimum level of acceptable performance, and the specification should be ratcheted up over time as new methods, new equipment, and new training offer that opportunity. Strive for

> Dr. Paul Barach (2006), an authority on patient safety, urges that more attention be paid to near misses.

the goal. Don't rest on meeting the spec. If each department just barely meets its spec, overall performance will be raggedy. Do better than spec.
- *Standardize.* Get everybody doing the tasks in the same way, every time. Pick the best way, of course. This is, invariably, a team effort and quite often illuminating. Reducing variability by standardizing minimizes the time that has to be allowed to cover the variability. That's progress already.
- *Measure and track.* Now that the process is standardized, simple tracking charts flag recognition of upsets in the system. Digging into the upsets may lead to corrections in the task. Reducing upsets necessarily means reducing variability, and as that source of variability goes down, the time allowance can go down. More progress.
- *Think about a breakthrough change.* Identify barriers that might be eligible for a breakthrough change. If you're going to make a change, logic says to go for a breakthrough. Make a change that is worth the bother. Measure the potential benefit in terms of patient flow. For instance, if the breakthrough

change increases bottleneck capacity, then more patients can flow through. If the breakthrough change eliminates some steps or moves steps out of a key time period, then the patient sees quicker treatment and, because every step is a potential source of variability, less time needs to be allowed.

A breakthrough is not always possible. Furthermore, an organization can only cope with a small number of changes at the same time that affect more than one department. So, some senior management involvement in deciding which break-throughs to pursue is going to be necessary. Breakthroughs involving more than one department should be given to a senior management sponsor who can monitor progress and pick up on policy changes that may be necessary.

- *Worry about communications.* Communication problems are common in healthcare. Poor handwriting is endemic; verbal orders are frequent and prone to misapprehension; jargon is opaque. Zillion-dollar computer systems may or may not eventually cure all this, but there are simple things to do in the meantime. See Chapter 13 for the Orange Form, a zero-cost communications breakthrough.

> If it's important to keep sup-positories out of ears, write your directions in common English.
>
> —From "Prescription Writing to Maximize Patient Safety," by Teichman and Caffee (2002)

- *Do a pilot.* Changes should always be tested by doing a pilot program, using measures and off-ramps. Pilots don't always work out, so be sure you can revert to the prior configuration.

- *Scale up.* Scaling up often reveals submerged barriers—barriers that didn't matter in the old system but interfere with the new one. These are only barriers, so they can be dealt with in turn. Tightening up the overall system takes away slack and requires, eventually, each affected unit to tighten up its own operations. This is perfectly normal.

- *Track and sustain.* To make sure that the improvement abides, track performance. Track value-added versus time in particu-lar. To sustain the improvement, encourage the work teams to strive toward the goal and not to rest on meeting the specification. Continuous improvement works, and it keeps everybody's head in the game, thinking not only about what is being done but also about how it is being done. Over time, continuous improvement is just as important as breakthrough improvement, and continuous improvement is always possible. Keep going toward the goal. Ratchet the specification up, over time as the process improves, to preclude backsliding.

THE SENIOR MANAGEMENT ROLE

Senior management sets the tone and clarifies everyone's thinking. Senior managers should be assigned to sponsor projects that cut across departmental lines. Senior management should stand ready to deal with compensation and contracting issues, because only senior management can. Compensation formulas need to reward patient flow, not departmental efficiency. The same goes for contracted services.

Healthcare workers are the brightest and best-educated workforce in the world and can learn the Lean skills quickly. Healthcare workers can figure things out for themselves, or senior management may wish to bring in specialists to accelerate the learning process. Be wary of consultants who claim to have healthcare competence but who can only produce factory experience. A hospital is not in the least like a factory, and you may be steered in entirely the wrong direction.

Here are two healthcare consultants who can produce ample healthcare success stories:

- Ed Popovich, president, Sterling Enterprises International, Inc., (561) 241-4978
- Richard Beaver, president, Six Sigma Connections, (412) 302-9900, www.sixsigmaconnections.org.

We have no connection with these consulting companies.

References

Barach, P. 2006. Lecture at the American Society for Quality meeting, Milwaukee, Wisconsin, July 14.

Frogue, J., D. Gratzer, T. Evans, and R. Teske. 2001. "Buyer Beware: Failure of the Single-Payer Healthcare." [Online article; retrieved 5/14/07.] The Heritage Foundation, lecture #702. www.heritage.org/Research/HealthCare/HL702.cfm.

Teichman, P. G., and A. E. Caffee. 2002. "Prescription Writing to Maximize Patient Safety." [Online article; retrieved 5/14/07.] www.aafp.org/fpm/20020700/27pres.html.

CHAPTER 3

Capacity, Backlogs, and Scheduling

With capacity matched to demand, either the patient or the provider will set the schedule. Which will it be?

MOVING BACKLOGS OFF THE MANAGEMENT TABLE

By backlog, we mean demand for the bottleneck service that is not yet satisfied.

For capacity planning, backlogs are a distraction. The strategic question is not whether there is a backlog, it is whether patients are entering the backlog at a faster or slower pace than they are leaving the backlog.

Consider a workable period of time—perhaps a week. Count the patients entering and leaving the backlog. Are more patients entering than leaving? If more are entering, then there is insufficient capacity. If fewer are entering, then there is too much capacity.

Given that most patients have some choice in healthcare providers, the balance between capacity and demand applies to all providers in the service region, aggregated together. If there is too much capacity, then there will be a battle for market share and prices will go down. The weakest competitors are going to be in big

> The existence of a backlog is not a signal to increase capacity. If the backlog is growing, add capacity. If the backlog is shrinking, cut capacity. Provide a surge in capacity to consume the backlog.

23

trouble. If there is too little capacity, then the provider who can increase patient flow through the existing system has a big advantage; its volume will go up and prices will stay up.

What about an existing backlog? Take extraordinary steps for a sufficient period of time to work off the backlog. Bring in temporary staff, bring in equipment on trucks, or transfer patients to providers outside the region. That will be doing the backlogged patients a favor and will eliminate the distraction.

WALK-IN SERVICE

Walk-in service provides maximum flexibility to the patient. However, if lots of patients walk in and find a crowded waiting room, then some will walk back out. Maybe they'll come back, maybe they won't.

Providers respond to this by setting up work schedules to match, roughly, the expected patient-arrival pattern over the day and week. That applies to maternity departments, emergency departments, walk-in clinics, and walk-in outpatient departments. What can the provider do to reduce waiting time? Two things: cut the processing time (improve patient flow) and improve patient information.

Cut Processing Time

If the processing time is zero, there can never be a queue. If the processing time is very short, there can only be a very short queue.

Consider a walk-in clinic with four doctors giving flu shots. Suppose six prospective patients walk in at the same time. Four go to a doctor immediately, and two wait. How long do they wait? They wait until two doctors are free. Suppose that's five minutes, and during that time ten more patients come into the clinic. How long will the last patient have to wait in queue? Fifteen minutes. If the processing time were cut to three minutes, then that last patient need only wait nine minutes. If the processing time were cut to two minutes, then that last patient need only wait six minutes. And, if the processing time were really zero, then that last patient would not have to wait at all because the 15 patients already in the queue would be finished in zero time.

Not many things can be done in zero time, but some can be done ahead of time and some can be done more quickly. Both of these options are fair game for the provider.

Inform the Patient

Traffic reporters on TV these days point at maps and tell the viewer how long the commute time is, right now. What can any viewer do with that information? Not much. Surely it would be better for that same traffic reporter to show a chart plotting typical commute times against times of day. Maybe present conditions can be put up as a line in a different color or as a flashing dot. If commuter traffic usually drops off after 9:30 a.m. and that information is shared with viewers, maybe some viewers can adjust their own schedule to stay out of the peak traffic period. Metropolitan traffic bureaus have that information. Why keep it a secret?

The same applies to any healthcare provider. Put the day's expected wait-time pattern up on the website and on an 800-number recorded message.

Informed patients, in their own interest, will tend to move to troughs in the traffic pattern if their other obligations allow.

BOOKED SERVICE

Booking fixed appointments reduces the queue of people in the waiting room while introducing other factors. One is that the patient may not show up, which wastes bottleneck capacity (and reduces revenue). Another is that the patient may show up late, which upsets the rest of the day's schedule. There are two things to consider for booked appointments: self-booking and small-flight booking.

Self-Booking

If your website allows patients to pick open time slots the way airlines allow passengers to pick flights and seats, then the patient is more apt to pick a time that will actually work from the patient's end. Furthermore, if lots of patients use the website, that open slot caused by Patient A's cancellation and rebooking is apt to be filled in by some other patient.

Airlines let passengers book a year ahead, collecting the money now. Having already collected the money, the airline doesn't care if the passenger shows up or not.

Healthcare providers can book a long way ahead, but they cannot collect the money. When the time comes, the patient may or may not show up, even if the patient self-booked. Too many things can intervene. The provider can make a pre-session telephone call or send a postcard to reconfirm, but that effort is not much different from the patient not having booked in advance.

A patient at the end of a long backlog queue has every incentive to book with several providers, hoping that one of them will call with an earlier opening. This compounds the difficulties of managing a backlog by encouraging bookings that will never come to pass. Self-booking works well if the booking applies to an early date, because the time selected is convenient for the patient. Self-booking, or any kind of booking, applied to a distant future date is unreliable. In other words, self-booking is a good complement to short-backlog operations.

Self-booking is not an antidote to long-backlog operations. This is one more reason to get rid of the backlog.

Small-Flight Booking

Consider a PET (positron emission tomography) scanner center. Consider that a PET scan takes perhaps half an hour, and assume that only one machine is available. For such a long processing time, walk-in service probably won't work, and some sort of booked appointments will be necessary to provide satisfactory patient service. On the other hand, if a booked patient is 20 minutes late, then the whole schedule is a mess for the rest of the day with lots of miffed patients. One way—not a good way—to deal with late-shows is to tell every patient to show up half-hour or an hour ahead of time. This merely constitutes group punishment. Let's consider another way.

Take process time to be 30 minutes. Book two patients for each 30-minute block of time—on the hour, say. Tell both to show up on the hour and that each of them will be out within an hour. One of the two will be pleased to be out early. If either of the two is late by as much as 29 minutes, the day's schedule still holds. This is called small-flight booking, with "flight" meaning a group of patients. This same policy works if there are two or three machines; just scale everything up.

This is an example of desensitizing the system to uncontrollable variability; in this case, the uncontrollable variability is the punctuality of the patient.

DIAL-UP SERVICE

People hate to wait on hold when they make telephone calls. There is no equivalent to a waiting room for telephone callers. So, capacity has to be matched quite precisely to demand. The easiest way to do that is to contract with a big call center, which can take calls for lots of clients at the same time and who can provide surge capacity. Indeed, the call-center's computer system does that automatically and pops the right screen up for the next available agent.

If there are reasons to keep the call-answering service in-house, then the capacity simply has to be made available to answer and serve nearly every call within a minute. A success story on this topic is in Chapter 5. Have friendly people, not machines, answer calls. No voice menus. Providing information on websites and on separate 800 numbers (say, dial 800-555-1345 for office hours) eliminates some calls. Separate 800 numbers are better than voice menus.

PREPROCESSING

Processing patient information before the patient's arrival reduces the duration of the visit, allows time for straightening out insurance or other payment difficulties, and generally goes in the right direction. Preprocessing can be done on a secure website. Preprocessing can be done by telephone call. Preprocessing can be done in a pre-meeting session.

Preprocessing calls attention to one matter—identification. How does the provider know that the person standing here is the person who was preprocessed? Identification is always an issue; preprocessing merely calls attention to the matter.

Patient Identification

Some healthcare providers issue ID cards. To these providers, a patient with an ID card and a PIN number is accepted as the patient belonging to the ID. That's fine if the patient shows up with the card and the PIN. What others are doing, across a range of industries, is using biometrics to provide trustworthy identification. That includes fingerprints, retina scans, and face prints. Some of these have big-brother connotation, deservedly or not.

One trustworthy biometric is thermal imaging of the back of the hand. No contact, so no contamination. It works right through a surgical glove, so it can be used for employees as well as for patients. It is used in hospitals, particularly in Japan, as well as in other industries (Biometrics.gov 2006).

This system, relying on the fact that the blood-vessel pattern on the back of the hand is as distinctive as a fingerprint, may be the healthcare identification system of the (near) future.

Patient ID comes up in three circumstances. We'll touch on each briefly.

Circumstance 1: Continuity of Care

A patient picked up at an accident scene, carried by ambulance to an emergency department, moved to surgery, moved to the intensive care unit, moved to postop, and eventually discharged needs to be tagged in some way so that drugs and other interventions given to the patient can be tracked, even if the name of the patient is unknown. If a number of patients are picked up at an accident scene, for instance, it's helpful to have a tag on each one so that as the patient is handed over at each stage, drugs already given will be known. Barcode bands work. RFID (radio frequency identification) works better, because no line of sight is required. Wristbands and stick-on plaques come with both these days.

> RFID is one tiny chip that acts as a computer and a radio, responding to queries by reporting its ID number. No battery is required, although a tiny battery extends the useful range.

Circumstance 2: History of Care

If the patient has previously been treated by the provider, then the provider will want to show that it applied good-faith effort to bring forward any information already in the files, such as patient allergies. If the patient is not in a condition to provide identification directly, then a passive biometric ID system fills the bill.

Circumstance 3: Actual Identification

Finally, it's a good idea if the actual name of the patient can be deduced so that family can be notified. If the patient is already known to the provider, as discussed in circumstance 2, then that information is probably at hand. If not, then an external database will be required.

Because Americans do not carry national ID cards, this is an open issue. Even if a driver's license comes to be the de facto national ID card, not everyone drives and not every driver carries this ID card at all times. Given Americans refusal to carry government-issued ID cards, it is unlikely that Americans will submit to a national registry of biometrics anytime soon.

What might work, though, is the voluntary contribution of biometric characteristics to private healthcare databases. The trend in health records is to keep the records in the patient's hands, away from providers and institutions. Maybe that will catch on. If so, someone may figure out a way for authorized healthcare providers to access a secure database of biometric identifiers. The data processing isn't hard, but getting everybody to see merit in identification for healthcare is not going to be easy.

Reference

Biometrics.gov. 2006. "Vascular Pattern Recognition." [Online information; retrieved 8/06.] www.biometrics.gov.

PART II

Basic Applications of The Lean Method

We apply the Lean Method to healthcare units that are simpler than a general hospital. We talk about barriers and bottlenecks, and we talk about ways of dealing with them. We include success stories.

CHAPTER 4

Simple Patient-Flow Examples

A wound center is a simple operation. Getting it to run as a business turns out to be not quite so simple.

THE WOUND CENTER

The flowchart for this wound clinic (see Figure 4.1) is about as simple as any flowchart could be. So why are we including it here? Because we wish to point out that treating the patient is not the only obligation of the care providers in this clinic. It is also necessary to log the facts of the treatment for billing.

Payers require that sufficient details of the treatment be written down to justify putting this patient's treatment into a degree-of-difficulty category. Payment is then made at a negotiated rate per category. Who keeps track of the treatment details? Who makes up the payment claim? Care providers are trained to provide care. They do not start out being trained in the intricacies of billing. Furthermore, those billing intricacies are not set in stone; they change rather frequently, so keeping up with those intricacies is an important task for somebody to fulfill.

Figure 4.1. Wound Center Flowchart

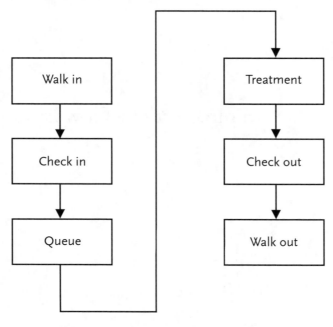

The person keeping up with payment issues is probably in the business office, but new information needs to reach the care providers and patient-record writers so that records will be generated in light of that new information.

To get this in hand, here's a way that is known to work:

Observe
1. Follow some representative patients all the way through the treatment process.
2. See how billing information is gathered and recorded.
3. Ask the workers where they get billing instructions.

Standardize
4. Get business-office people and caregivers in a room to make a flowchart.

5. Invite workable solutions to complexities that arise.
6. Settle on one standard way of doing everything.
7. Do a pilot program to smoke out any unforeseen barriers.
8. Retrain as necessary, and issue new documents as necessary.

Track
9. Do a tracking chart on a case mix. Chapter 18 offers a figure of merit for a case mix that is easy to track.
10. Do a tracking chart on changes in billing rules that are likely to trigger an increase in billing exceptions while people adjust.

In a small unit such as a wound center, it may be appropriate to train the caregivers themselves, rather than the medical-record specialists, to create the record for each case as it is going along. Perhaps the entries into the record should be checked by a second qualified person (we encourage paired workers for everything), and promptly while the facts are still at hand.

THE MRI CENTER

This application focuses on improving the upstream stage of an MRI center.

Let's consider a freestanding MRI center so that some basics of patient flow can be seen in a simple setting.

The MRI center has a bottleneck—the MRI machine. Adding capacity to the center would require a major capital-dollar outlay to upgrade or add MRI machines. Because in this case the bottleneck is obvious, management will be alert to all upsets within the bottleneck and will be attentive to all proposals to improve patient flow within the bottleneck. Indeed, it may be said that the bottleneck will be managing the manager.

There are activities upstream and downstream that merit attention and that, if handled successfully, will enhance patient flow by making sure a patient is ready when the MRI machine is ready and by completing the patient's care once through the machine. These things are less apt to cry out for the manager's attention; therefore, they require positive attention by the manager and reinforcement by senior management.

The flowchart (see Figure 4.2) shows quite a number of actions upstream of the bottleneck. Perhaps some of these can be done ahead of time so that they do not have to be done at the time of treatment. At least two of the upstream tasks—the interview and the coaching—might vary quite a bit from patient to patient and therefore constitute a source of variability in the total process time. If those highly variable steps can be done ahead of time, that will both shorten the list of things to be done and reduce the variability on treatment day. Reducing variability upstream is always good.

Figure 4.2. MRI Center Basic Flowchart

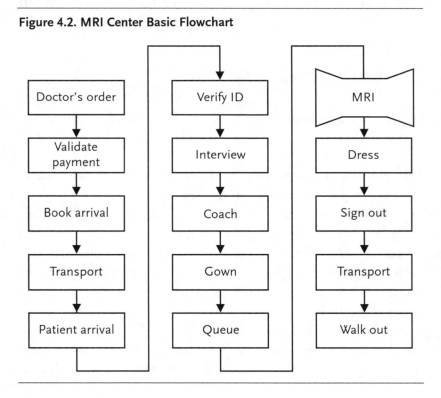

Reducing variability anywhere is always good. Reducing variability upstream is important because the only way to deal with it, if it cannot be reduced, is to bring patients in extra early. That is not apt to please patients.

On the other hand, the most efficient way to do the interview might be to do it on treatment day. Doing it ahead of time might be less efficient. What should management do?

This provides a simple example of the Lean Method versus a cost-reduction method. Lean says, do as many as possible of the upstream things ahead of time without regard to efficiency. The Lean objective is not to reduce costs; it is to improve patient flow. The steps that can be done ahead of time, in most cases, appear to be those shown in Figure 4.3.

Figure 4.3. MRI Pretreatment Session Flowchart

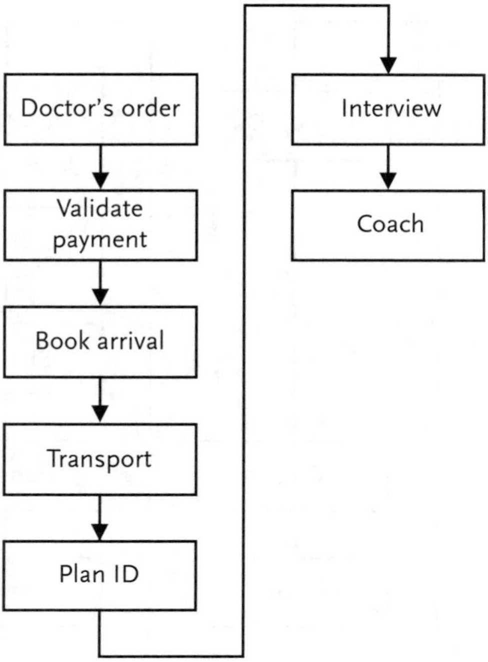

A pretreatment session might be done at the patient's residence or perhaps over the telephone. The pretreatment session provides an opportunity for an extensive interview, if appropriate, and a lengthy coaching session so that the patient will be less apt to balk at treatment time. This might be supplemented by information on the center's website or a mailed video presentation on MRI in general, what to expect, why this MRI center is better than others, and any other reminders such as how to call the center if a change in schedule needs to be made. The patient or family member can be instructed on what identification documents to bring and on other administrative matters. Then, when the patient arrives for treatment, the treatment-day upstream tasks are reduced and the flowchart for treatment day looks like the one shown in Figure 4.4.

Figure 4.4. MRI Reduced Upstream Flowchart

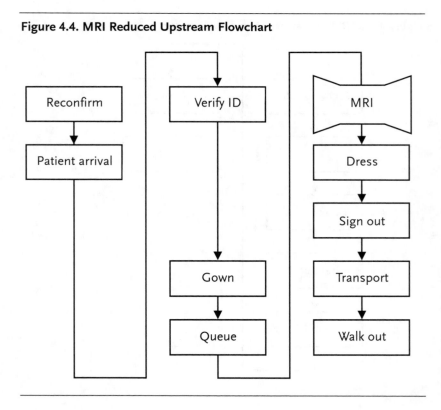

There will still be some uncontrollable upstream variability, such as the patient's diligence in getting there on time. This uncontrollable variability puts the MRI center at some risk of running out of patients, leaving the machine idle, and not producing revenue. The center's management will want to do something to hedge against late-shows, in addition to reminder telephone calls.

Here's one to try. Suppose the MRI run-time is 20 minutes. Book two patients at 9:00 a.m., the next two at 9:40 a.m., and so on. That is booking in flights of two. Tell the patients making up each flight to be present 15 minutes before MRI time to allow for signing in and putting on a gown, and then say that the treatment will be done within 40 minutes of MRI time. That provides a hedge against one or the other patient being late by as much as 19 minutes. It does not put an undue wait on either patient if both are on time.

A Success Story

Here's a real-life MRI barrier story; see the MRI center's patient flowchart in Figure 4.5. A hospital purchased an upgrade to its MRI system, and the vendor assured the hospital that seven more patients would be processed every shift. The hospital found, instead, that no

Figure 4.5. MRI Floor Plan and Patient Flow

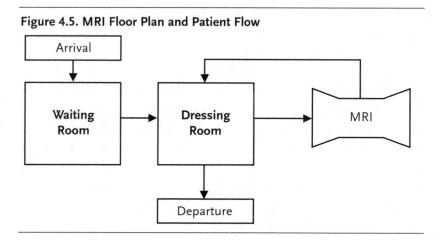

additional patients were being processed, vendor assurances to the contrary notwithstanding. Careful observation revealed that the dressing room was congested so that an increased number of incoming patients were blocked from getting changed into gowns, and the MRI machine was left waiting.

Does this mean the bottleneck moved? No, the bottleneck is still the MRI machine. The undersized dressing room was a barrier—a self-imposed limit—that could be easily removed by management's act of rebuilding the dressing room. In this case, the barrier was not intentional, but then barriers never are. They are discovered, just like this one was.

Unanticipated barriers often arise when a revised system scales up after the pilot program. These are called "submerged barriers." As they appear, fix them. If another one appears, fix that too. Barriers always lie within management's range of action.

THE CANCER CARE CLINIC

This application focuses on getting the interested parties to see the big picture.

Consider a freestanding cancer clinic. The bottleneck is the number of oncologists on duty to provide treatment. The flowchart (see Figure 4.6) is about the same as for the MRI center previously discussed, with a "prior session" to gather information, coach the patient, organize transport, and plan an identification system.

Identification gets extra consideration here. The cancer treatment can be lethal, and therefore the center has to make very, very sure that the patient is identified to a high degree of certainty. Many patients cannot testify to their own identity. The patients will probably come for several treatments over a period of time, and they are probably not coming from a hospital where they would be wearing a hospital bracelet. If they are accompanied by family, that would help, because the family member can provide the identity. If they are accompanied by the van driver of a long-term-care facility, that's not much help.

Figure 4.6. Cancer Clinic Flowchart

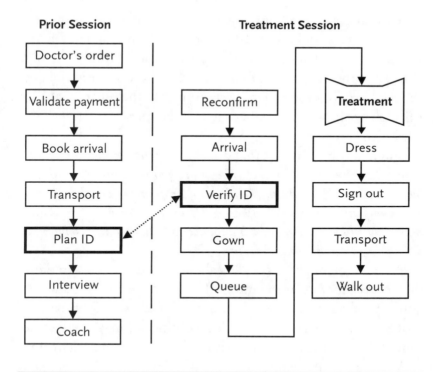

Part of the work to be done in the preparatory phase, then, is to take steps to ensure identity. Tattoos go in and out of fashion.

A subcutaneous radio chip in the forearm works and is now being used in some circumstances. A photo, with permission from the patient, helps.

Some hospitals issue ID cards. Other industries use fingerprint scans, retina scans, and face recognition. Some hospitals use back-of-the hand scans. There are lots of options.

> Invisible tattoos are now used on dairy animals, replacing ear tags. The invisible tattoos act as RFID devices (see Jones 2007).

> VeriChip[1] received FDA approval for subcutaneous ID chips in October 2004. VeriChip and others also make paste-on ID chips.

An Example

Here's a cancer care center story. The upstream process at the center was proving to be unpredictable, with some patients being held up so long that the oncologists were idle. With the oncologists being the bottleneck, that's bad; the idea is to keep the bottleneck busy. To observe what was going on, the nurses made up a flowchart, in which one barrier was the nurse's interview and assessment process.

You may ask, Why was that done? *That's the standard procedure.* Why? *Requirement.* Whose? *The Joint Commission.* Would you please show me? *Well, maybe it's not a written requirement, but it's an important professional responsibility we have as nurses to do this interview and assessment, and if we don't do that, then there's not much we're doing that amounts to nursing.*

Ah ha! One might expect "local optimization" to mean doing the necessary work in the most efficient way. Here, nurses were doing *extra* work because they thought it necessary for their own professional self-regard. It's still local optimization—doing something for a local reason that does not contribute to patient flow.

What to do? If the nurses were ordered to stop doing that task, workplace morale would be at risk. What to do? After some consideration, other work of high professional standing was found for the nurses to do instead. As it happened, that other work was billable separately, so total revenue went up a little. But revenue enhancement was not the driver—improving patient flow was. That new professional work is teaching patients beforehand about the treatment and about follow-up home care.

The Lean Method generated this favorable result by leading the participants to consider why each step is being done and whether it could be moved out of the treatment-day flow. Issues were brought to the surface, and creative solutions were found. People are good problem solvers, once the problem is squarely put.

Note

1. VeriChip Corporation is a subsidiary of Applied Digital Corporation, www.verichipcorp.com.

Reference

Jones, K. C. 2007. "Cattle Call: Startup Touts Invisible RFID Ink." *Information Week* (January 15).

CHAPTER 5

Call Center:
A Success Story

Callers get prompt service now because the call center has applied observation and standardization. No breakthrough required.

BACKGROUND

The Army Medical Command sustains a healthy and medically protected force. It provides care to soldiers, their family, and other beneficiaries around the world (some 5.9 million persons in total) using 30 major medical facilities and numerous clinics. A typical day brings 37,000 clinic visits, 6,300 radiology procedures, 82,000 pharmacy procedures, 52,000 laboratory procedures, 60 births, and 25,000 dentist visits.

The Fort Hood Army base in Texas, which has more than 100,000 enrollees, has one central call center that books appointments for six primary care clinics and 60 specialized clinics. The center handles as many as 10,000 calls per week. It is the largest call center in the Army Medical Command and employs civilian call agents.

The call center has a typical automatic call distribution (ACD) telephone system that keeps callers on hold; feeds calls to available agents; and keeps basic statistics on calls attempted, completed, rerouted, and abandoned. Agents follow scripts for each call, and because various callers require different information from the agent, agents have to follow a total of 30 distinct call scripts. Scripts are incorporated into the agent's computer screen.

OBSERVATION PHASE

Getting patient input was easy; there were lots of complaints. Average hold times were at least three minutes, and 26 percent of all callers and 50 percent of busy-hour callers hung up and tried again later (which meant they were in queue at least twice). Previous attempts to improve service had not gotten anywhere.

Observation was applied to the telephone system. It came to light that there were two pools of calls—one from on-base callers and one from outside callers. On-base callers were automatically getting lower priority. Furthermore, there were two queues, and it was possible for a caller to wait in one queue only to get dumped at the back of the other queue!

Observation was applied to the time it takes to complete the appointment transaction. Talk-time was found to be 126 seconds on average. Agents did not do any write-up work between calls. Value was being added during those 126 seconds. Not much value was being added at any other time during the whole appointment-booking process.

SETTING A GOAL AND A SPECIFICATION

The goal is what an ideal system would deliver. The goal is to answer every call before the first ring. The practical specification, going in the direction of that goal, was set thusly: Answer 95 percent of all calls in any half-hour, including the busy half-hour, within 90 seconds.

STANDARDIZATION PHASE

The first standardization action was to get rid of the two levels of call priority and the two queues so that all callers were treated the same, with one pool of callers and one queue. The 30 scripts were scrutinized and rewritten to get the necessary information from the caller while being polite and cutting down on nonessential chatter. Agents were encouraged to stay with the script so that every call was treated in a standard way.

Agent staffing was adjusted to match the historical hour-by-hour traffic. Attention was paid to the fact that "agent at station" is not the same as "agent ready for next call" when setting the staffing schedule. For example, it was found that an agent needs about 15 minutes at the beginning of a shift to log in and set up the station for use. Previously, agents had been scheduled to start at 0700h (7:00 a.m.), and the telephone lines were opened at the same moment. This meant that everything was backed up by 15 minutes before the first call was answered. Agents are now scheduled to start work 15 minutes before they are expected to take calls.

Some additional changes were made. Agent desks were rearranged so that an agent can transit the work area without interfering with other agents. Scripts were rearranged so that the availability of an appointment slot was confirmed before taking patient data; this saved only a few seconds per average call, but it reduced the patient's annoyance level substantially.

BREAKTHROUGH

No breakthrough change was required to achieve satisfactory performance.

TRACKING AND CONTINUING TO IMPROVE

The existing ACD reports facilitate tracking. Tracking allows continuous adjustments in work schedules as calling habits change. The accumulating traffic history provides a planning basis for Fort Hood and for comparable call centers throughout the Army Medical Command.

PROGRESS TO-DATE

The following table shows prior and current states of affairs at this call center.

Parameter	Old System	New System
Calls per week	10,000	8,000
Calls abandoned, busy hour	50 percent	18 percent
Calls abandoned, full day	26 percent	4 percent
Calls answered in 15 seconds	42 percent	77 percent
Calls answered in 90 seconds	65 percent	93 percent

Note that the number of raw calls per week has gone down. That's because fewer patients now find it necessary to make two or three attempts to make an appointment.

MANAGEMENT MESSAGE

Breakthroughs are not always necessary. New equipment is not always necessary. In this case and in many others, it is sufficient to observe, standardize, and adjust operations to get substantial improvements. Getting the appointment is part of patient flow, because the patient thinks it is.

Note

We are pleased to acknowledge Mark Hernandez, senior managed care/access to care specialist in the AMEDD OneStaff TRICARE Division, for his special contributions to this chapter.

CHAPTER 6

Outpatient Laboratory:
A Success Story

Empowering patients to do their own registration cuts cycle time dramatically.

BACKGROUND

Heritage Valley Health System[1] has an outpatient lab to which patients go to have blood drawn and other tests performed. The center used to have a waiting room with 40 chairs. Patients booked appointments by telephone. Upon arrival at the waiting room, each patient registered at the desk, gave the usual information, and awaited service. Average door-to-door patient time was 1 hour and 10 minutes.

OBSERVATION

A process-improvement team observed these operations, gathered patient-traffic data, and set about streamlining the operation to improve the patient flow.

As seen in Figure 6.1, there are only two steps in the door-to-door patient flow—registration and treatment. Neither of these could be construed to be a bottleneck, because more registration desks and registrars could be added and more technicians and specialists could be added. These are barriers, not a bottleneck. The door-to-door time of 70 minutes appeared to be a large multiple of the minutes required to draw blood. This looked like a potential for breakthrough improvement, and the eye is drawn to the registration step. Adding a registration desk would not constitute a breakthrough, but new technology might.

External benchmarking revealed that airports were changing from agent check-in to passenger self–check-in at kiosks. The passenger books travel on the airline's website, which gathers any necessary information, and then the passenger goes to a kiosk upon arriving at the airport and enters flight information. That's it. Transaction times drop markedly and queues shrink.

Figure 6.1. Outpatient Laboratory: Before and After

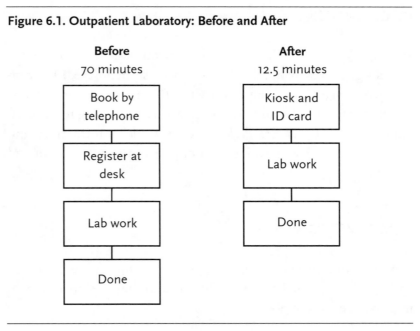

Going Lean: Busting Barriers to Patient Flow

Heritage Valley issues patient ID "Care Cards," which have a bar-code on the back. These are like grocery store frequent-shopper cards. Anyone can sign up for a Care Card on the hospital's web-site. They're free and do not create any obligation to the hospital or the prospective patient. The process-improvement team used the Care Card as a building block and bought the self-service kiosk solution from a vendor for the waiting room.

BREAKTHROUGH

The arriving patient now walks up to a kiosk, scans the Care Card, enters her birth date for verification and security, and uses the kiosk touch screen to select the service desired or to see a scheduled test. The kiosk feeds the data to the care-provider's computer screen. Kiosk time averages about 90 seconds. Armed with the information already provided, care providers can then move more efficiently from patient to patient. Door-to-door patient time is down from 70 minutes to 12.5 minutes on average (see Figure 6.1). That saves nearly an hour out of the average patient day. Nothing has changed in the medical service provided; the process redesign simply eliminated nonproductive time.

Replacing the desk registration with the kiosk is an example of the fact that there can be no queue if the process time is zero. The kiosk time isn't quite zero, but it goes much farther in that direction than a registration desk could possibly do. The telephone registration is no longer needed. With the automated check-in, walk-in service is just fine. The waiting room has been reduced from 40 chairs to 25 chairs.

Heritage Valley is looking to further refine the process to cut the door-to-door time a little more. Perhaps fewer chairs in the waiting room will help. That is to say, the health system will not rest on the breakthrough improvement but will now seek continuous (non-breakthrough) improvements over time.

Outpatient labs at other facilities can use Heritage Valley as an external benchmark and a source of inspiration. This model can be expected to work for any treatment process involving only a few minutes of actual treatment time.

Note

1. Hospitals are in Sewickley and Beaver, Pennsylvania; see www.hvhs.org. Management at Heritage Valley provided the information in this chapter.

CHAPTER 7

Back Pain Clinic:
A Success Story

Standardizing cuts painful waiting time by a factor of ten.

BACKGROUND

Virginia Mason Medical Center in Seattle has a spine clinic. Starbucks is a large employer in the Seattle area. A number of Starbucks employees develop lower-back pain and go to the medical center for treatment (Fuhrmans 2007).

Dr. Robert Mecklenburg, Virginia Mason's chief of medicine, called on Ms. Annette King, benefits director for Starbucks, to elicit concerns, if any, about the service being provided by the medical center to Starbucks employees.

Ms. King directed Dr. Mecklenburg's attention to the incidence of back pain, which was costing Starbucks lost workdays and money.

OBSERVATION

Dr. Mecklenburg met with the spine clinic staff. A number of patient records were reviewed. It became clear that there was no standard diagnostic process. Patients might first be sent for an x-ray and given pain pills. If the condition persisted, then another visit to the doctor was ordered for additional analysis, often including an MRI exam, and physical therapy was commonly prescribed.

Indeed, the point of the multistep diagnosis was to sort out which patients had minor cases and which had more serious cases. For many patients, a month went by from the first call for an appointment to the time physical therapy began.

STANDARDIZED PROCESS

The spine clinic staff, with input from the employer, developed an evidence-based standard process for uncomplicated back pain. This process includes same-day access. Having done so, they agreed that because most patients are eventually given physical therapy, with only the exceptional patient getting some other treatment, the standard process ought to start with physical therapy in mind.

A patient first sees a physical therapist, then a doctor. If the physical therapist and the doctor agree that the patient's condition warrants physical therapy, physical therapy is prescribed, and treatment begins immediately. As long as physical therapy improves the condition, no further treatment is prescribed.

If not, or if exigent conditions are evident at the first doctor's visit, then other therapies would be pursued. See Figure 7.1 to see the difference between the old and the new patient flow.

BREAKTHROUGH

Patients now get appointments within a day. Most patients go into physical therapy that same day or shortly thereafter. The exceptional patient is seen on a longer schedule by specialists.

Figure 7.1. Spine Clinic Patient Flow: Old and New

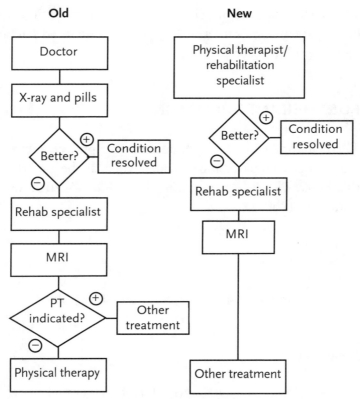

Source: Flowchart used with permission from Virginia Mason Medical Center, Seattle, Washington.

OUTCOME

Most patients are into therapy within three days rather than 30 days. Treatment begins with a physical therapist at the first visit, not after a trip to the doctor, to x-ray, and to the MRI center. That's a ten-fold reduction in the time a typical patient has to wait, and suffer, until treatment begins. Because most patients are being seen only once by spine-center specialists, physicians have more time to spend on serious cases that need more advanced therapies.

CAPACITY

The newly designed spine clinic was able to offer five times the number of patient appointments, at a 13 percent reduced staff and with 18 percent less space.

FURTHER INFORMATION

There are other interesting aspects to this project, including gain sharing between payer and provider, which are beyond the scope of this book. Please read the *Wall Street Journal* article by Vanessa Fuhrmans (2007).

Note

Management at Virginia Mason provided additional information in this chapter.

Reference

Fuhrmans, V. 2007. "A Novel Plan Helps Hospital Wean Itself Off Pricey Tests." *Wall Street Journal* (January 17).

CHAPTER 8

Women's Center:
A Success Story

Boca Raton Community Hospital reduced the cycle time from 13 weeks to one day for a woman coming in for a mammogram, being told more tests were needed, and eventually getting a disposition. Thirteen weeks of anxiety reduced to one day, with treatment starting within the week. That's improving patient flow.

BACKGROUND

Boca Raton Community Hospital is a 394-bed community hospital with a women's center that puts emphasis on mammography for detecting breast cancer. The center performs more than 20,000 mammograms, 9,000 diagnostic mammograms, 4,000 ultrasounds, 3,000 MRIs, 4,000 bone density exams, and 2,000 biopsies. More than 350 cancers were detected in 2005. More than 42,000 procedures of all kinds were provided that year.

Dr. Kathy Schilling, a radiologist who practices at the center, has joined with mathematician Dr. Heinz-Otto Peitgen to develop and apply fractal mathematics to imaging for early breast-tumor detection. The fractal concept is that, in many cases, close-in views of an image have the same appearance as faraway views of the same image. Dr. Schilling and her associates found that the fractal concept applies to the blood vessels around breast tumors, so visualization of vascular flow and flow disturbances is a sensitive indicator of tumor presence. This permits earlier detection, when tumors are still small and easier to treat. This also permits detection of tumors occluded by other tumors or by dense material between the tumor and the camera. The benefit of this research is greatest when the patient has early access to screening and there is minimal holdup time between mammographic imaging and MRI imaging. Protracted delays vitiate the early-detection advantage.

The women's center had upgraded from analog to digital mammography (replacing nine analog units with three digital units), expecting the digital units to be able to process more patients per hour. Although the digital units performed to the manufacturer's specifications, the performance of the center did not seem to be satisfactory. Patients were unhappy with long waits; staff members were unhappy with the lack of service improvement; and there was a general feeling that things were not as they might be. The center's management and staff were pleased to have any help and were open to new ideas from others as well as from themselves. Cooperation was extended, and the Enterprise Excellence project was launched.

Enterprise Excellence

In March 2004, CEO Dr. Gary Strack of Boca Raton Community Hospital in Florida created the Enterprise Excellence department. Staff members were assigned and trained in process-improvement methods. Becky Southern and Mark Viau[1] took up the women's center as their first major project. Dr. Strack appointed a senior manager (himself) to sponsor the project and to meet weekly with the project teams.

PHASE ONE: OBSERVE, STANDARDIZE, STREAMLINE

The starting point is always to figure out what the baseline is. In this case, what are the queue times? How many patients are being processed? What's the no-show ratio? Are some patients jumping the queue, thereby annoying all the others? What happens, and what is supposed to happen? Observing from a chair in the waiting room soon revealed that patients were upset when appointments were not honored, even if the delay was only 15 minutes. Observing the technologists at work revealed that there was little standardization.

The center had just purchased digital-examination equipment, which kept records online. However, to have prior-years' films for comparison, the physical films had to be fetched from an off-site storage facility, which required either a three-day notice or a special trip to the storage facility. Each patient visit was booked as a separate event, so a patient who needed a second exam made a new appointment, which meant the patient's total treatment time stretched out (see Figure 8.1). The waiting time between visits turned out to be awfully long, particularly considering the anxiety the patient must be enduring while waiting for the next appointment, not knowing and fearing that she may have cancer.

Figure 8.1. Old Scheduling Model: Typical Patient Experience

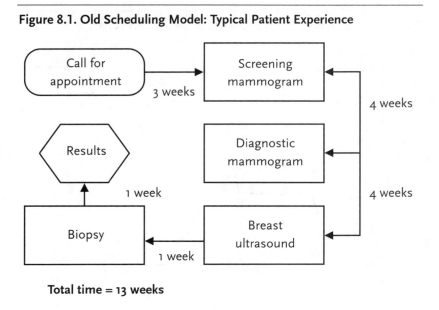

Total time = 13 weeks

Figure 8.2 is a value-added versus time chart, based on the booking lead times in effect under the old flow at the center, starting with the patient's arrival for the screening exam.

The First Visit

Fetching records from the off-site storage facility was introducing delay and variability into the preparation for a patient's first visit. What to do?

Mark Viau, who has extensive experience with radiology, facilitated the team that looked at the matter systematically. He proposed that the hospital-floor space presently used to store x-ray films for the medical center's radiology department be swapped with the center's off-site space. Space requirements matched well enough, and the traffic in film-fetching favored the women's center. The departments

---

Figure 8.2. Old Patient Flow: Value-Added Versus Time Chart

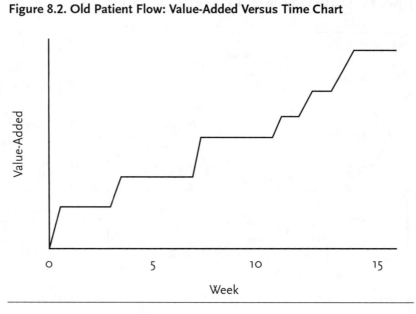

agreed, and senior management okayed the unbudgeted cost to swap the storage.

Participative Creativity

The team, having learned a great deal by looking at the first step in the process, decided to draw a diagram to portray the interaction of the interested parties. The result is seen in Figure 8.3.

Everybody seemed to be interacting with everybody else. To the team, that meant having to be careful in proposing any changes, to make sure that all involved parties know what's going on and have a chance to speak up before things happened.

Figure 8.3. Interaction of Interested Parties

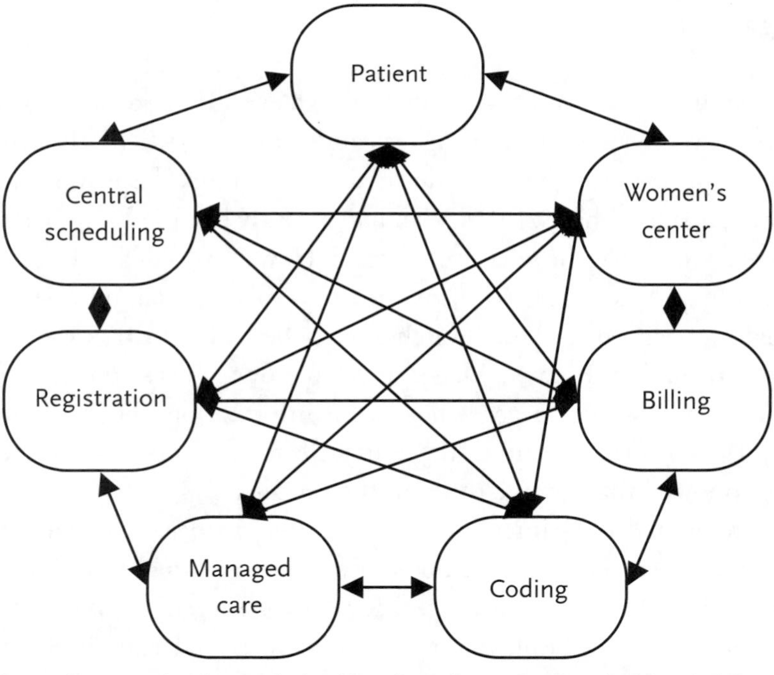

Source: Data used with permission from Boca Raton Community Hospital, Boca Raton, Florida.

Then the team observed how workers did their work. Getting a common, standardized way of doing the tasks had never been considered important before, so long as the patients were cared for and the radiologists were presented with high-quality images. The team leaders explained that standardization was necessary so that variability would be reduced and so that baseline quantification would mean something. Process variability is controllable and should be controlled. There would still be variability from patient to patient, and those uncontrollable sources of variability would be observed after the process came to be controlled. The uncontrollable variability would be dealt with as part of the process redesign, to allow ample time for care, to allow for contingencies, and to provide for recognizing upsets when they happen. After a creative discussion, a common, detailed, flowchart was developed and agreed to by all those involved.

Tagging Whales

With hundreds of patients coming through every day, tracking every patient seemed to be a daunting task and would overwhelm the center's resources. So, the team decided to do things the way whale watchers track whales. Mark Viau had recently been to Hawaii and there learned that the whales offshore in Hawaii would later be seen offshore in Alaska. How did anyone know this? A small number of whales are tagged, and then watchers elsewhere find the tags and log the information. Because whales travel in groups, it is not necessary to tag every whale to get some useful information about all the whales. With that in mind, the team selected a sample of patients and followed that sample through the process.

The actual run-times for the screening exam were observed. Previously, screenings were booked for five minutes; actual run-time was about 6.5 minutes for most screening patients. Diagnostics were booked for 30 minutes; actual run-time was about 15 minutes for most diagnostic patients. But the average time was not the only characteristic of interest. How variable were the treatment times? Were the times bunched around the average, or did they vary all over the lot? Figure 8.4 shows the sampled distribution of session times.

Looking at this chart, a reasonable time allocation would be 15 minutes. Some patients would take more time, and these would tend to cause a backup in the waiting room. Further observation revealed that the few patients who took a lot of run-time were usually patients in wheelchairs who needed special assistance. This might have been factored into the scheduling, although the team decided that it would take some time to build this issue into the database and left it for a future date.

Still, there is some variability, and an occasional patient would need 30 minutes. What should be done to offset that variability? The team decided that the impact of the occasional 30-minute patient could be minimized by having one single patient queue for the three machines, with the next patient going to the first available

Figure 8.4. Session-Times Distribution

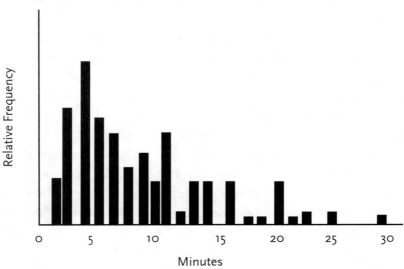

Source: Data used with permission from Boca Raton Community Hospital, Boca Raton, Florida.

machine. This is the way banks queue customers these days. Grocery stores, on the other hand, have separate queues for each checkout counter. Single queue seemed to the team to be the better choice here.

Little thought reveals that the single queue, while delayed by a 30-minute patient, accelerates when a 5-minute patient goes through. The single queue allows these long and short cases to average out to keep a smooth flow going.

Optimized, Yes, But How?

The preexisting process was designed by bright people and had evolved over a long period of time, ever since the hospital had been doing mammograms. It was clearly optimized by some measure, for some good purpose. A combination of looking at how things were actually done and interviewing the staff revealed that the preexisting system was purposefully designed and optimized with one idea in mind—to maximize the productivity of the radiologist.

To get to this optimum, screening patients were processed one at a time and then the images were viewed by the radiologist one after the other, in a batch. Diagnostic patients were processed one at a time, and then the images were reviewed in a batch. The radiologist could then read through the two batches of films, or digital images, quite quickly with minimum distraction.

On the basis of that design rule, the process was well designed. Perhaps that is the best design rule. Is the radiology staff working dawn to dusk reading images? Are radiologists in short supply? Are there professional rules or some sort of regulation at play? Do radiologists insist that things be done this way? Is there evidence that the most limiting resource is the radiology staff?

Looking at the tagged-whale results and following up with other observations, the conclusion was no; the limiting resource was the number of machines. More machines would increase production, even with the same staff. The machine count constituted a barrier that could be removed by buying another machine, albeit at a substantial but not impossible cost.

PHASE TWO: OPTIMIZE FOR MAXIMUM PATIENT FLOW

The team decided to redesign the process so that each patient would be provided same-day processing. One visit. This would be less efficient for the radiologists, who would no longer be doing batch processing.

A few practicalities now intrude. One is payment. Before the day of the appointment, it is necessary to verify insurance coverage or apply hospital rules for self-pay patients. The payment question pops up again at each stage, if the paying insurance company requires that a new authorization be obtained at each stage. Even if additional authorizations are routinely averred, they take time and may require more than a phone call. Hospital senior management made the policy decision to give the best care and to haggle with payers after the fact.

It was learned that many family physicians believed it their professional responsibility to counsel the patient before the biopsy, given the serious implications. That meant an extra day or so in the process to allow for the films and radiologist's report to be shipped, electronically, to the family doctor and then for the doctor to meet with the patient. Given that the point is to provide the best medical care, this judgment call is appropriate, and if the family doctor wanted to do this face-to-face with the patient, so be it.

Based on the information in hand, it was determined that the booking schedule should be 15 minutes. This was enough time for 95 percent of the cases, and with three machines and next-available-machine utilization, the occasional extra-long case did not create a backlog of patients.

Pilot Test

The purpose of any pilot program is to try things out before betting the farm. When the team was confident enough to pilot the patient-focused flow, the team planned a pilot, including provisions for off-ramps just in case things didn't work out. By definition, provision to revert to the prior system is planned into any pilot.

A pilot can work with a fraction of the total traffic or with all the traffic for a block of time. The team chose the latter and picked October 24 through November 8, 2005. On October 24, however, Hurricane Wilma struck. So much for best laid plans. After the hurricane and the cleanup, the pilot began again and was successful. All essential points of the new flow were verified. No submerged barriers arose.

The radiologists were satisfied that proper care was being given. No operational glitches came to light. The patient queue seemed to be running smoothly. Patients said they were happy with their care.

Changeover

After a review by the team, the oversight board, and other interested parties, the women's center changed over to the new flow. For instance, the typical schedule for a patient booked on a Tuesday became this:

Tuesday: Screening and diagnostic exams
Wednesday: Family doctor meeting (if patient needs a biopsy)
Thursday: Biopsy
Friday: Treatment planning with the multidisciplinary clinic

On occasion, when the family doctor wishes it, the biopsy is performed during the first visit as well, cutting Wednesday and Thursday out of the process. One-day service is then achieved.

Catch Up

Patients who were partway through the process on the old system were given individual attention to get their total work completed.

PHASE THREE: IMPROVE

The team presented management with solid data to show that revenue would increase by adding one mammography machine, bringing the count up from three to four. All other resources were adequate to serve the additional traffic.

Management authorized the capital outlay for the machine—some $400,000 dollars—based on the business-case analysis and the expected return on investment.

The multidisciplinary clinic medical staff, while exuding pleasure that patients were getting to them weeks earlier than they did under the old system, asked if an MRI could be squeezed in after the biopsy without delaying the overall schedule. Affirmative. MRIs are now being booked for Day 4, which is Friday in the earlier sequence that started on Tuesday, so that the MRI results are available to the multidisciplinary clinic medical staff by the time the patient gets there the following Tuesday.

PRESENT SITUATION

With the new flow standardized, and with standard block times allocated, the capacity of the system is established and documented. Departures from the standard flow are readily seen and responded to. Management has solid business data for any follow-up decisions that may be required. Patients are happy. Demand is up. Technologists are happy. Radiologists are happy. The business office is happy. Senior management is happy.

There have been a number of second-order benefits, too. For instance, a gown costs more than a dollar; the new flow reduces the number of gowns consumed over the year. Other consumables are reduced, too. These are not major contributors to the hospital's bottom line, but they repay some costs—such as the cost of relocating the film archives—and go in the right direction. Still, the objective was not to reduce cost. The objective was to improve patient care by improving patient flow.

Workload and Schedule

The committed capacity is 100 patients per day. The physical capacity is about 113 patients per day. The demand is about 135 patients per day. By holding back a modest fraction of the physical capacity (13 percent), the women's center management has some surge capacity to catch up in case of upset—another hurricane, say, or a machine breakdown. By providing less capacity than the market would fill, management is making a prudent, informed business decision.

Patients commonly book, when present for a session, for a follow-up exam a year after. About three-quarters of the capacity is booked this way. These patients get pre-appointment telephone calls to revalidate insurance and straighten out other such matters. Boca Raton, like many Florida cities, has a much higher winter population than summer population. Capacity planning has to take this into account because, unlike the hotels, the hospital does not charge winter rates. Yet.

New Center Design

A new women's center is contemplated, partly on its merits and partly because a whole new hospital is contemplated. As part of this study, some information useful to the design of the new women's center came to light. That is the foot-traffic pattern—the route walked by a patient and a technologist during the course of a treatment. When plotted over a sketch of the floor plan, these traffic patterns are often called spaghetti diagrams. Figures 8.5 and 8.6 are sample spaghetti diagrams.

Figure 8.5. Spaghetti Map for Patients

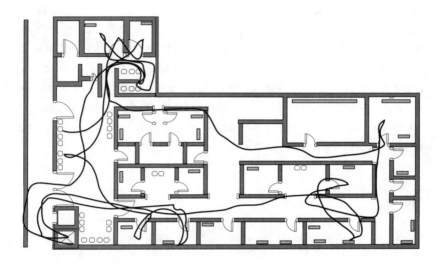

Figure 8.6. Spaghetti Map for Technologists

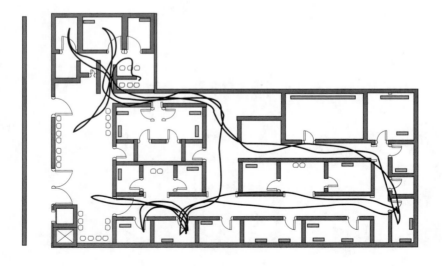

It seems likely that the original design of the current building did not involve this much spaghetti. Over the years, technology changed, machines changed, additional functionality was inserted, and things were shoehorned in. These are unavoidable in any dynamic field of medical practice. Even so, the next floor plan and machine layout may benefit from the present spaghetti-tracking information, which is available to the architects who will design the new center. As part of the new design process, estimates of the future spaghetti can be drawn as well, just to make sure things are going in the "less spaghetti" direction.

Note

1. We are pleased to acknowledge Becky Southern and Mark Viau, who were the leaders for the project reported in this chapter, for their special contributions.

PART III

COMPLEX APPLICATIONS OF THE LEAN METHOD

Complex systems are complex. While gains can be made by applying the Lean Method to discrete units within a complex system, such as a general hospital, greater gains can be made by dealing with the whole. Identify the bottleneck and the barriers, apply the Lean Method, and improve patient flow. Specific recommendations are included. Success stories are included.

CHAPTER 9

The Lean General Hospital

Patients move from unit to unit. Units tend to optimize locally. Getting to patient-flow optimization requires overcoming local optimization.

BACKGROUND

Putting Lean into the operations of a general hospital is a matter of putting the same principles to work in a multistep patient treatment. The organization is more complex, and there is a strong tendency for each department to seek its own local maximum level of efficiency. While efficiency is a good idea, local efficiency upstream and downstream of the bottleneck tends to work against maximum patient flow.

In the next several chapters, we will look into departmental operations with a view toward moving local management in the direction of better patient flow, even at the expense of reduced local efficiency. It's a question of global optimization (for the patient) versus local optimization (for the department).

We'll provide success stories, too. We will also make specific recommendations that deal with specific needs of high-patient-flow hospitals. These are based on real-life experience and success. For those who prefer to read the last page of a book first, we will summarize later those recommendations given here for the convenience of the reader.

First, let's pin down the bottleneck. All Lean analysis starts with the bottleneck.

THE BOTTLENECK

The bottleneck in almost every hospital is the inpatient bed count. Maximum turnover of inpatient beds makes best use of the bottleneck and maximizes patient flow. There are upstream units, such as clinics and emergency departments. There are downstream units, such as rehabilitation units. Some of these may be part of the same hospital; others may be independent, but they are still involved.

Traditionally, each unit has organized its work to maximize its own efficiency. Optimizing for patient flow means giving up a little of that efficiency, unit by unit. While this may be done willingly in many cases, in others it may require changes in compensation bases or new contract terms.

SPECIFIC RECOMMENDATIONS

On Inpatient-Intake Control

Someone needs to know what patients are available for admission and what beds are going to be free, hour by hour. Someone needs to apply the hospital's admissions policies on self-pay admissions. This "someone" needs to be positioned just upstream of the bottleneck so that live information about available beds and live information about available admission candidates is applied promptly, consistently, and in conformance with hospital policy.

We recommend that a "patient-flow control desk"[1] be created and charged with this responsibility. All inpatient admissions go through this desk. No bypasses. This desk is the information node. Management needs information to manage. This desk is where it's at. We'll develop this idea in Chapter 12.

On Observation-Patient Placement

Observation patients are different from emergency department patients and from regular inpatient patients. The observation patient needs attention for hours, rarely for days, and doesn't fit into the inpatient routine. Payment for observation is closer to the emergency department model, with additional payment for additional services, than to the regular inpatient payment scheme of fixed payment per admission DRG (diagnosis-related group).

We recommend that a separate unit be established for observation patients, with this unit being geared for hours of stay, not days of stay, and with administrative support for the per-item billing required for these patients.

On Hospitalists

Hospitalists are medical doctors who specialize as attending physicians. Hospitalists make hospital operations management easier because the number of individual doctors to deal with goes down by a large factor. It is easier to get a modest number of doctors to conform to a new process than it is to get a large number to conform. The hospitalist specialization lends itself to timely bedside detection of upsets in the patient's progress, prompt adjustment of care, and timely discharge. This seems to be a good idea all around.

Hospitalists join service line managers and case managers in having a longitudinal interest in the patient and in having less of the task orientation that others involved in the patient's care necessarily and appropriately have. This longitudinal interest promotes patient flow.

Note

1. Some hospitals use the term "intake control desk."

CHAPTER 10

Emergency Department

The emergency department is upstream of the bottleneck. Its role is to provide a flow of qualified patients to become inpatients while providing emergency care.

BACKGROUND

The emergency department is always interesting because so much goes on there. The patients are rarely scheduled; they just show up. Traffic varies greatly and is subject to sharp peaks triggered by external events. Every patient presents a unique set of needs. While these factors can be estimated in advance from prior experience, they are not controllable. The emergency department needs to be designed to cope with all these variabilities.

Most hospitals believe that a large and well-regarded emergency department acts as an attractor of patients for surgery, inpatient, and follow-on services, which generate revenue. The emergency department is a gateway to the hospital. This is entirely consistent with the emergency department being an upstream function, feeding patients to the bottleneck—the bottleneck being the hospital's inpatient bed count.

The emergency department is obliged to treat patients without consideration of the patient's ability to pay. The emergency department needs to be governed by policies covering

1. holdup time policy versus patient service,
2. uncompensated care beyond the obligated level, and
3. internal operating practices.

PATIENT FLOW THROUGH THE EMERGENCY DEPARTMENT

Some patients flow through the emergency department to become inpatients. They may become inpatients at this hospital, but they may be transferred to become patients at another hospital. Let's look at a basic flowchart for these patients (see Figure 10.1).

There are two boxes on this chart that attract our attention—the waiting room box and the holdup box. Patients in the waiting room have a low expectation of service and accept that more urgent cases will bump into the queue ahead of them. Quicker service would be

Figure 10.1. Emergency Department to Inpatient Flow

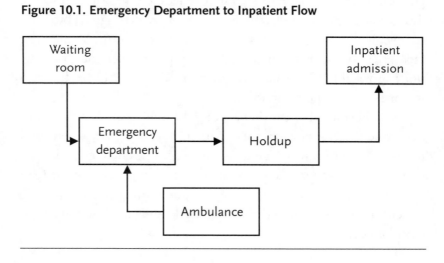

Going Lean: Busting Barriers to Patient Flow

welcome, but there is no expectation of prompt service. It's not that way when patients get to the holdup box on the flowchart. Patients held up, waiting for inpatient admission, have a much higher expectation of prompt attention. The emergency department of Boca Raton Community Hospital[1] in Florida found the correlation in Figure 10.2.

No surprise there. Long holdup times mean poor patient satisfaction scores. But why is the holdup time not under better control? There's nothing new here—patients have been transferring this way since emergency departments were invented.

Let's look at the bottleneck for insight. The bottleneck is not in the emergency department itself; the bottleneck is the inpatient bed count. If the inpatient department has empty beds at the moment the patient is declared ready for transfer, then the holdup time is near zero because the patient can be transferred immediately. If the inpatient department has no empty beds at that moment, then the patient will be held up until a bed becomes available.

Figure 10.2. Patient Satisfaction Versus Emergency Department Holdup Time

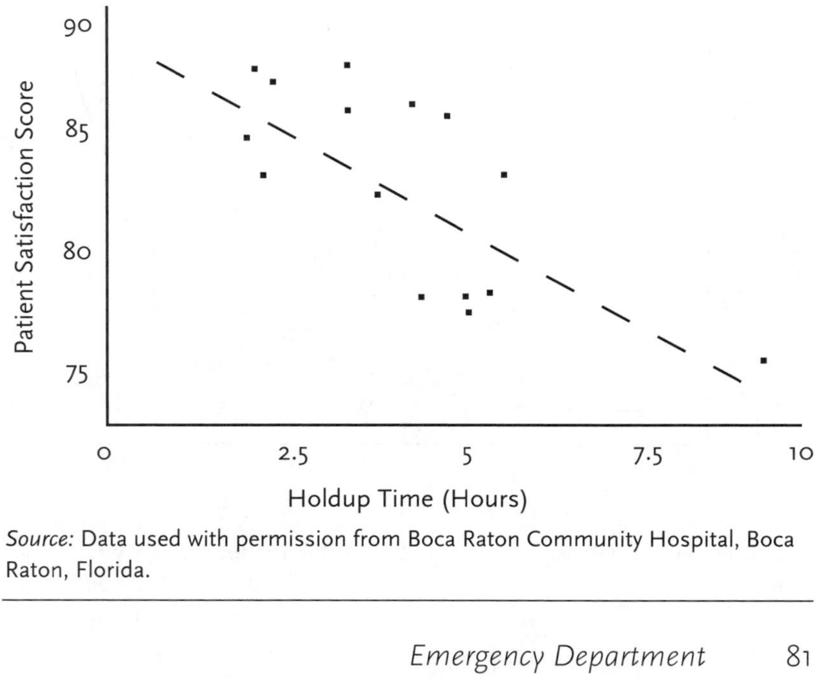

Source: Data used with permission from Boca Raton Community Hospital, Boca Raton, Florida.

Given that emergency patients present themselves at all hours of the day and night, while inpatient departments tend to discharge patients in daylight hours, it stands to reason that the likelihood of having an empty bed at a particular moment depends on how close the inpatient department is to full occupancy. How close to full occupancy does a hospital have to be before the holdup times get out of hand? Data for this have been recorded by the emergency department of Boca Raton Community Hospital in 2005 (see Figure 10.3).

Boca Raton Community Hospital sees the holdup times shoot up when the occupancy rate gets much beyond 80 percent to 85 percent. Let's think about that. At 80 percent occupancy, there must be dozens of beds empty at the time the daily census is taken. Yet, patients are waiting hours for transfer. What can the emergency department do about this? After all, it's the emergency department that gets blamed for this, and with the most to gain, the emergency

Figure 10.3. Patient Holdup Versus Hospital Census

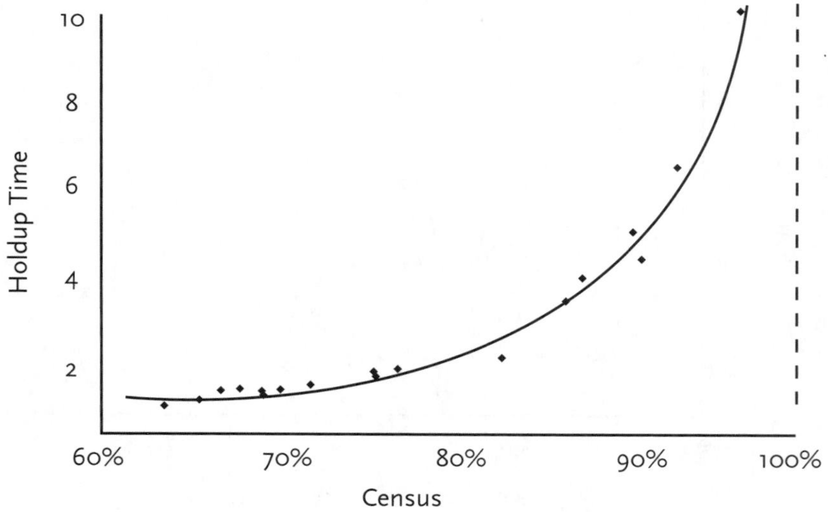

Source: Data used with permission from Boca Raton Community Hospital, Boca Raton, Florida.

department will be the keenest to get holdup times down and patient satisfaction up. What can the emergency department do?

Nothing.

Adding emergency department capacity moves patients more rapidly from "waiting room" to "holdup." Reducing emergency department capacity reduces the number of patients in holdup, but only by increasing the number of patients in the waiting room. Neither of those sound promising, so emergency department capacity should be set on medical grounds—matching capacity to number of patients with urgent needs—without consideration of holdup time.

The best way to reduce the number of patients in holdup is to figure out how to move those patients into the hospital by improving things on the hospital side of the holdup. Short of that, is there nothing the emergency department can do? Well, there are two things, and both are routinely done. One is to reduce the number of patients coming in the door by diverting ambulances to another hospital. The other is to transfer patients from holdup to another hospital.

Diversion of ambulances is commonly done when the emergency department's capacity to deal immediately with urgent cases is swamped. Would it be appropriate to divert ambulances solely to improve patient satisfaction with holdup times, which for these patients is a few steps down the flowchart? That is to say, divert patients who are not in holdup to prevent building up the patient count in holdup.

Transfer of patients to other hospitals is commonly done when available inpatient capacity is zero. For instance, the particular patient needs intensive care and this hospital's ICU is full. Would it be appropriate to transfer patients to other hospitals solely to improve patient satisfaction by reducing holdup time?

Competition for Inpatient Beds

While the emergency department patient is waiting for an inpatient bed, other competition for that bed arises from direct admissions, from nonelective surgery, and from elective surgery. While direct admissions can be refused and elective surgery can be postponed, common sense says that all of these input streams need to be managed according to consistent rules, or the result will be holdups in all of these streams and the same sort of (low) patient satisfaction levels will apply everywhere.

What to Do

Work closely with the inpatient patient-flow control desk to provide timely updates on immediate and projected need. (See the patient diversion success story later in this chapter.)

Increasing inpatient capacity may be very difficult or expensive to do. That's why it's called the bottleneck. The best overall strategy is surely to run at a high inpatient occupancy level to make the best use of the bottleneck. Find consistent policies that support that goal while providing good medical care and patient service throughout. Consistent policies would recognize that there is no significant policy difference between postponing or refusing to schedule an elective surgery and diverting an ambulance to another hospital. The same goes for transferring a patient from holdup to another hospital. All of these recognize that the hospital has limits on the level of service it can provide to its patients and that providing the expected level of patient satisfaction may be more important than incremental patient counts. Good patient satisfaction pushes demand up.

Diversion and transfer policies need not be entirely reactive. Based on traffic history, the next-day emergency department demand can be forecast, reasonably, for each period of the day. The elective surgery schedule is known for the following day and the scheduled direct admissions are known for the following day, hour by hour. Armed with the present inpatient occupancy level, a workable forecast can be made for the following day and a diversion plan can be set up. Diversions can be ordered or put on standby.

Transfer planning can be initiated so that cooperating hospitals can be on notice. This can be done before the actual patients are known by name.

Applying a modicum of next-day forecasting to emergency department surges goes in the direction of better patient satisfaction and merely anticipates what would be done the next day when the surges are already there. Putting all patients on polite notice that they may have to be transferred if no local bed is available goes in the right direction and takes the edge off as a patient dissatisfier.

Notice that not much of this forward planning can be done by the emergency department alone because it has no control over elective surgery or inpatient operations. Therefore, the hospital may wish to empower a neutral agent to trigger such policies (see the patient diversion success story at the end of this chapter).

The best course of action is to reduce length of inpatient stay, speed up inpatient discharges, and turn the inpatient beds around rapidly to make beds ready for the next patient and to expedite the information flow about bed demand and bed availability. Reducing occupancy causes the holdup time to drop rapidly, according to Figure 10.3. That's the nice thing about nonlinear curves. Even though they hurt a lot going one way, they help a lot going the other way.

OPERATIONS

While emergency departments have no control over the condition of the patients coming in or the time of day the patients come in, emergency departments do have control over their own operations (see the door-to-balloon success story at the end of this chapter).

It's a good idea to have standard procedures for each type of patient—with all teams doing things the same way—and to apply robust ways of doing the basic tasks. If operational standards are followed, then variability in outcomes cannot be laid to variability in process. That's good; it eliminates one source of variability. Applying robust methods is not hard. The fundamentals can be stated simply as follows:

1. Tag the patient, and maintain the tagging throughout the stay in the emergency department.
2. Echo verbal instructions to close the loop.

3. Use the NATO phonetic alphabet or any phonetic alphabet you like better.
4. Work in pairs—one observing and reminding the other.
5. Design tasks to be more likely to succeed than to fail, to permit any inadvertent error to be seen on the spot, and to permit immediate remediation.
6. Log actions, drugs, and materials immediately.

Patients who are picked up by ambulance should be tagged at the scene, and the same tag should be retained as long as the patient is in the emergency department realm. The patient may have been given drugs at the scene or en route, or there may be more than one patient coming from the same scene. Tagging goes in the right direction. Wristband barcodes are good, but the active RFID tags now entering wider use are better (see Chapter 3). An active RFID tag has a little battery to give a boost to its radio signal, so the tag can be read through the patient's body, on the other side of the bed, and out of the line of sight. Using the same tagging system takes a little planning and coordination with ambulance services—all for a good cause.

Generating the log of services and consumables in real time provides the most reliable basis for toting up the bill for services. How to do this when the patient needs all hands? One method is to assign a clerk to keep the log in real time. Another is to create an audio record on the fly. Both are more robust than asking a nurse to recreate the record from memory later on.

Minor Needs

Emergency departments often provide a nurse practitioner to deal with minor needs, such as rewrapping a bandage or cutting off a ring. This frees up the emergency physicians to deal with more serious matters, shortens the queue for the patients needing only minor treatment, and goes in the direction of improving patient satisfaction.

When the patient comes in the door, a triage nurse considers the patient's condition and, if appropriate, directs the patient to the nurse practitioner's queue. It is important that this assignment be enforced. If the patient needing only minor care is left to decide whether to go to the nurse practitioner or to go to the emergency department per se, the patient will choose the one that looks to have the shorter queue. This is familiar to anyone who shops in supermarkets with less-than-10-items counters. The shopper with just a few items picks freely among all the checkout counters and picks the shortest queue. The next shopper with a large order then has to wait, and the likelihood is that the small-order counter queue will dry up from time to time. It's the same here. If the patient has a free choice, then traffic can only move away from the nurse practitioner, which defeats the purpose of providing the minor-needs queue in the first place.

This is known as the "iron law of stratified services" (Barry and Smith 2005). This law applies elsewhere in the hospital, too. If a nurse has non-nurse assistants, then the non-nurse assistants tend to be idle and the nurse tends to be overworked (Weinberg 2003).

Note

1. See www.brch.com. Information in this chapter was provided by Ed Popovich, vice president of Enterprise Excellence, Boca Raton Community Hospital, November 2006.

References

Barry, R. F., and A. C. Smith. 2005. *The Manager's Guide to Six Sigma in Healthcare*. Milwaukee, WI: ASQ Quality Press.

Weinberg, D. B. 2003. *Code Green*. Ithaca, NY: Cornell University Press.

Patient Diversion: A Success Story

An emergency department solved its diversion (lost business) problem by solving its admissions problem.

The emergency department at the Western Pennsylvania Hospital—Forbes Regional Campus (part of West Penn Allegheny Health System) solved its diversion (lost business) problem by solving its admission problem.

For about 60 hours a month, during the summer of 2005, ambulances were being diverted away from the emergency department at Forbes because the department was full. About 200 would-be patients were lost to other hospitals; the patients were inconvenienced; and somebody was paying for extra ambulance rides.

Because the emergency department is a gateway to Forbes's other services, the hospital was forgoing about $3 million per year in revenue. Forbes's emergency department had 16 beds at that time.

OBSERVATION

A self-selected, self-actuating team decided to fix things. The team started properly, by observing what was going on, not just in the emergency department but in every related department. First, the team observed the emergency department. Then, the team observed for 12 hours on each hospital floor. The team took lots and lots of notes about operations, bed locations, patient movements from department to department, and who did things quickly and who did things less quickly. The team filled up notebooks and filled up white boards with ideas, diagrams, arrows, boxes, and note clouds.

ANALYSIS

Who knows when a bed is empty? Who knows how many beds are empty and where they are? What is the discharge process, not in the emergency department but in other parts of the hospital? Why does that take so long?

The team found that the intake process, starting when an emergency department patient gets to an inpatient department, takes a nurse one hour. That's information gathering and certainly necessary, but is that information already known someplace else? Can some of it be standardized? How about some productivity tools?

FOCUS

The team decided that there were two key issues that the team might be able to deal with. One was timely information about beds. The other was setting a trigger for team action. That is to say, when should the team jump in and do something extra?

PILOT

The team decided that the bed information was simply not known by any single person, so the team established twice-daily, all-parties meetings (brief ones last not more than 10 or 15 minutes) to exchange information on beds available at that moment and the bed forecast for the rest of the day. These meetings included someone from each floor unit, someone from housekeeping, someone from the emergency department, someone from surgery, and anyone else who might be an information source. The point was to tell everybody where the available beds are at that very moment and where they are apt to materialize during the next half-day.

Eventually, the team decided that in addition to these meetings, one person needed to know everything and to be the repository of the information, so the team appointed one nurse to be the patient-flow controller. The team decided, after much thought, that any patient on a gurney in the emergency department hallway was one too many. The goal was set to zero. The first such patient was declared to be the "trigger." That trigger convoked a bedside meeting of concerned parties to figure out what could be done to place that patient, right now.

OUTCOME

Ambulance diversions are a thing of the past at Forbes. Forbes's emergency department treated 40,000 patients within a year with its same 16 beds—quite a substantial number for a suburban hospital with only 16 emergency department beds. Emergency department traffic is up by more than 1,000 patients. Revenue previously forgone is now captured.

NEXT ROUND

In those twice-daily meetings, the team now addresses contingency planning. What would we do if there were a sudden spike in emergency department traffic sometime in the next 12 hours? What buffers can we establish? Where do we have some flexibility?

As an endorsement of the good work done, the Forbes board has allocated capital to expand the emergency department from 16 beds to 25 beds.

REMARKS

Of the two key changes instituted by Forbes, one had nothing to do with the emergency department per se; it had to do with admissions and discharges from inpatient departments. The emergency department is at the mercy of these other departments; this was noted earlier in the chapter.

The other key change—the trigger—is revealing. The Forbes team asked itself, what is our goal for the number of heldup patients waiting for an inpatient bed? *Zero.* Well, if our goal is zero, when do we start taking extraordinary action? *With the first patient held up.* This shows empathy for patients and a keen sense of mission.

The substance of this breakthrough is an improved system of communications. In this case, the improvement amounts to reverting to the oldest of communication modalities—standing face to face and exchanging information.

Note

Management at Western Pennsylvania Hospital—Forbes Regional Campus provided information in this chapter.

Door-to-Balloon: A Success Story

Cut the time from door-to-angioplasty by doing steps in parallel.

BACKGROUND

The national standard for emergency care of patients with a heart-related concern is for angioplasty balloon treatments to be given within 90 minutes from the time the patient comes in the door. This is called the door-to-cath rule or the door-to-balloon rule. While this can be approached by requiring a cardiologist to be near at hand 24/7, an interesting and successful approach has been taken by Heritage Valley Health System.

Figure 10.4 is a flowchart of the traditional door-to-balloon process.

Figure 10.4. Door-to-Balloon Process: Before Improvement

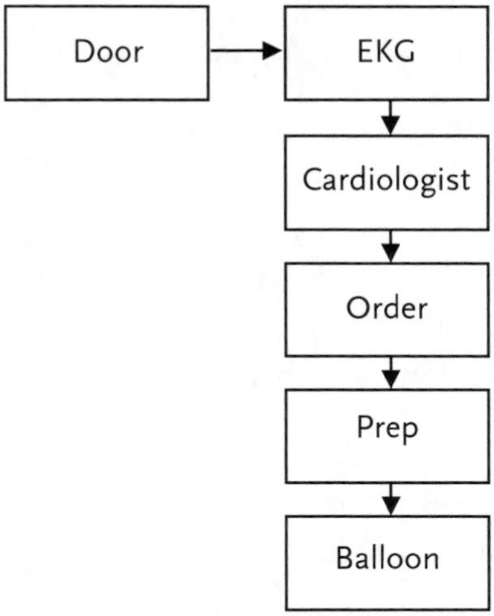

As shown in the figure, the patient declaring chest pains arrives in the emergency department (ED). The patient is put on an ED bed, and an EKG (electrocardiogram) is administered; the standard calls for this to be done within ten minutes of the patient's arrival. The ED doctor examines the patient and the EKG, concluding that a cardiac condition exists. The doctor brings in a cardiologist for consultation. The cardiologist orders an angioplasty. The patient is prepared and moved to the heart-catheterization room, and the cardiologist performs the balloon angioplasty.

If the cardiologist is already on hand, then allowing ten minutes for the EKG, ten minutes for the first diagnosis, 30 minutes to prep and move the patient, and 30 minutes to do the procedure leaves ten minutes for the consultation. That is to say, ten minutes for the cardiologist to receive word, go to bedside, confirm the diagnosis, and make the order.

Perhaps the other steps can be compressed a little to allow more minutes for the cardiologist to reach bedside, but it would still be a close call. If the cardiologist needs to be called in from outside the hospital, squeezing a few minutes out of the other steps probably isn't going to be enough.

BREAKTHROUGH CHANGE

Heritage Valley dealt with this process in a different way—moving the cardiology consultation out of the direct flow and into a parallel position, freeing up lots of time. Figure 10.5 shows the improved door-to-balloon process at Heritage Valley.

As seen in the figure, the one change in the flowchart is this: the ED doctor does the initial diagnosis and orders the catheterization procedure if needed. The cardiologist is notified of the order and that the patient is being prepped. The

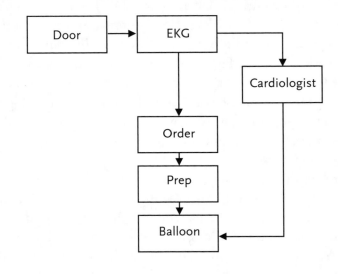

Figure 10.5. Door-to-Balloon Process: After Improvement

cardiologist arrives at the catheterization bed, confirms the diagnosis, and proceeds with the treatment.

Using the same 90-minute standard as before, the cardiologist now has 40 minutes to arrive, which is an improvement over the ten minutes allowed in the traditional process. This eliminates compressing any other steps.

REMARKS

This is an interesting example of management challenging the process. Who's allowed to order something? Why exactly is that? Isn't the patient better served if [insert your own ideas here]? Is the present system a matter of habit, or is there a substantial reason for doing things the way they are being done?

In the new flow, the order is given by the ED doctor rather than a cardiologist. There is some chance of a false-positive; that is to say, the doctor may order the treatment for a particular patient when a cardiologist may not. At this writing, Heritage Valley has not experienced any false-positives. That is encouraging, although the likelihood is that eventually there will be some small number of false-positives.

In the old flow, any false-positives would have been generated by a cardiologist. The likelihood would presumably be lower in that case, because the cardiologist is the specialist. The proper comparison is the differential in false-positive rates, ED doctor versus cardiologist. The false-negative opportunities are the same between the two processes, so false-negatives do not figure into any consideration of the relative merits of the two flows.

With a shorter door-to-balloon time, the patient ultimately benefits.

NOTE

1. Hospitals are in Sewickley and Beaver, Pennsylvania (see www.hvhs.org). Management at Heritage Valley provided information in this chapter.

CHAPTER 11

Laboratories

Labs and other support services are often on the critical patient care path. Changing operations from batch to flow helps the patient, even if it is less efficient for that lab.

ROLE IN PATIENT FLOW

Laboratories, left to themselves, tend to optimize their work to be the most efficient. That's good.

No, that's bad. Labs should not be efficient on their own; they should be efficient contributors to patient flow. Rather than focusing on the task, labs should focus on lab-report flow.

When focusing on the task, labs will find that work can be done more efficiently in batches. But batching necessarily extends the time to complete the average report, because the average sample has to wait until enough samples are in hand to make up the next batch. Doing each sample on its own (or if that's not practical, doing samples in small batches) improves the flow because the average sample has to wait less time. It may well be less efficient to do flow rather than batch. Okay, it's less efficient for the lab; it may take more labor and take more supplies. Even so, those are trivial issues compared to the value of patient flow.

Labs are very likely to be on the patient's critical path because the attending physician needs the lab reports to finalize the diagnosis and to confirm progress.

COMMUNICATIONS

Tracking

Order a package to be delivered by UPS or FedEx, and on their website you can check the location of your package, from door to door, at every stage of the flow. Send a blood sample to the lab, and how do you know where it is, if it got lost, and how far through the process it is?

UPS, FedEx, and other shippers let customers see their internal tracking information. The key is that these companies initially wanted this information for themselves—for their internal operational control—but later decided to make it open to customers. Giving customers web-browser access to the same information cut down enormously on telephone calls from anxious customers.

Does your hospital have this information for its own internal tracking? Why not? There's plenty of barcode technology available to log the progress of each lab specimen as it moves through the system. RFID is even better, and it's handier to use.

Reporting

A pathology lab supervisor in a large hospital told us that he had become interested in the hospital's process improvement program, and that led him to look again at his day-to-day operations. One element was a reporting system that logged the tissue analysis by patient and that sent the report to the accounting department. The supervisor was moved to walk over to the accounting department to find out who read the report once it got there and what was done with the data. Nothing. No one read the report. No one did anything with his data.

The accounting system had been changed some long time before, and the new accounting system rejected all of his input because it didn't conform to the "new" input format. The accounting manager explained that a variance report had been going back to the pathology lab every month showing that large variance. The accounting manager then pointed out to the lab supervisor where to look—in the back pages of a large computer printout.

That was a variance to the accounting manager. It was wasted effort to the lab supervisor. It was unbilled work to senior management, if any senior manager had even known about it.

Closing the Loop

Communications really does require closing the loop. This applies to all communications everywhere, and it certainly applies to labs and other service departments. Others really do need to know the status.

Closing the loop means a little more than sending back a report that the other party cannot understand; it means closing the loop in a way that both parties have a meeting of the mind so that problems are recognized and dealt with. That applies to bloodwork that might have gotten lost, and it applies to accounting reports that need to be understood by line managers.

SMALL-BATCH LABORATORY OPERATIONS

The most efficient mode of operations is to wait until a batch of work big enough to fill up the machine is to be done, and then do it all at once. That's the most efficient for the lab itself. Is it the most efficient for each patient? Well, no.

The first patient to be handled as part of the next batch has to wait longer than the next, and so on. If the batch processing time is a few minutes, then it won't matter. If the batch processing time is counted in hours, then the queuing time does matter. Running a smaller batch, not a full batch, reduces the queuing time for the patients who get into the small batch. Running more, smaller batches is favorable to patient flow even when unfavorable to laboratory efficiency. Who decides? That's ultimately a question for senior management.

Pathology Lab with Small Batches: A Success Story

A change from big-batch processing to small-batch processing cut turnaround time in half.

Here's an example reported by the UPMC Shadyside Hospital pathology lab (PRHI 2004).

The tissue sample arrives at the pathology lab.

1. Pathology assistants examine the tissue in the gross room and extract samples.
2. The samples are batched and processed in a machine to infuse formalin.
3. The samples go to histology, where they are embedded with paraffin wax.
4. The samples are chilled, sliced, and placed on blocks.
5. The blocks are stained in another machine.
6. The stained blocks go to a pathologist for analysis and reporting.

The observed turnaround time was 24 to 48 hours. The process improvement team asked, "If we make 24 hours sometimes, why not all the time?"

Each step in the process was deemed necessary, and the lab had a low error rate. There was no need for corrective action at the task level, only an improvement in completion time at the system level. Further observation revealed that while large tissues needed to be in the first machine for 12 hours, smaller tissues required only three hours. Additional observations revealed that the tissue blocks, once chilled, needed to be kept cold, and the existing handling equipment was designed for chilling a group of 10 to 20 tissue blocks. There was no equipment on hand to keep just one tissue block chilled.

BARRIERS OVERCOME

The team determined rather quickly that they faced at least four barriers in trying to get every sample done within 24 hours.

1. At least one new equipment item was required to handle a single chilled block.
2. The work schedule in each group was organized to do batches.
3. The layout of the room was convenient for batches but maybe not for singles.
4. If no batching were done, then the capacity of the lab was not known.

The team went to work. A hobbyist contributed a single-block chilled carrier, which uses an ice chamber as a way to keep the tissue-block surface cool. The team reorganized the workstations. Tinkering began.

The team decided to start each morning with a three-hour run of the first machine to treat small tissues, which were immediately handed over to the next station. Then a batch of larger tissues was run for 12 hours. Eventually the team decided to alternate large-tissue and small-tissue batches. The second workstation, which received a small batch, did its work and handed over each block one at a time to the third station. So the blocks were progressively de-batched as they proceeded through the lab. Completion times of 24 hours were achieved for all cases. Mission accomplished.

In the new model, the same tasks are performed at each stage. Each stage works the same fraction of the day as before. The difference is that in the old model, the workers at the later stages had to wait twice a day for a batch of blocks. Now they wait for shorter times for single blocks. More start-stop. If they get behind for some reason, they can catch up by filling in those "stop" periods. Final delivery is smoothed out.

Now, the mode of production for the pathology lab is to work on blocks as soon as any are available for work. That's called *push*.

A SUBMERGED BARRIER REVEALED AND OVERCOME

As you have now guessed, there is another mode of production called *pull*.

While making these changes, the team addressed a source of annoyance in the old mode of operation, which was the ordering of supplies. Previously, a histotechnologist went around once a week and took orders for supplies. This took eight person-hours per week. In the new mode, anybody wishing supplies hangs an order card on a hook; the cards are gathered up at the end of the day, which takes just a few minutes; and supply orders are placed every day. This has improved employee satisfaction, reduced stock-outs and emergency orders, and eliminated the source of annoyance.

> The supply-reorder model here is similar to the Japanese *Kanban* system. No supplies are pulled until an order card is presented. *Kanban* is Japanese for punched card.

This is another example of small batching or de-batching. The new supply-ordering system is a *pull* model; no supplies are pulled from stores until needed.

SHARING LESSONS LEARNED

The team later consulted with Detroit-based Henry Ford Healthcare System, a 900-bed system where the de-batching ideas were put to work. There, the old practice was to make up a batch of 60 blocks for the staining machine. That was changed from waiting for enough blocks to make a full batch to starting a new batch based on the clock; every 20 minutes the machine is started, using whatever blocks happened to be on hand. This increased the number of same-day biopsies, completed within nine hours, from 81 percent to 93 percent (PRHI 2006).

Note

PRHI and management at UPMC Shadyside Hospital laboratory provided the information in this chapter.

References

Pittsburgh Regional Health Initiative (PRHI). 2004. [Online newsletter, August; retrieved 9/12/06.] www.prhi.org.

———. 2006. [Online newsletter, April; retrieved 9/12/06.] www.prhi.org.

CHAPTER 12

Admissions

OBSERVATION VERSUS INPATIENT ADMISSION

Before we take up the wider question of how to manage hospital admissions, let's consider the narrower but still instructive matter of "admit for observation" versus "admit as inpatient."

The insurance payment for observation status is much lower than the insurance payment for inpatient status. Some hospitals refuse to admit any patient for observation. On the other hand, insurance payment for observation status is like insurance payment for outpatient treatment, à la carte. If a CT (computer tomography) scan for an observation patient is ordered, insurance pays for it. If a CT scan for an inpatient is ordered, insurance does not pay for it.[1]

Operationally, an observation ward is like an emergency department, where it is expected that the patient's presence will be brief. An observation stay is perhaps two hours. That doesn't match up very well with an inpatient ward, which is geared to overnight stays and three meals a day. Should a general hospital have an observation ward, or should a general hospital put observation patients in beds with the inpatient population? Because of the difference in operational habit, it would seem that a separate ward for observation patients is preferred. The size of the separate ward can be determined by historical and projected demand, including the expected, short duration of each observation stay. The observation ward would be run like the emergency department with an expectation of short stays. There are published standards for determining whether a patient fits observation status or inpatient status (see McKesson 2006; Milliman Care Guidelines 2006).

Let's consider a physician who writes an order to admit the patient as inpatient, for observation, or for observation with cardiac monitoring telemetry. Figure 12.1 is the basic flow. The physician decides what service the patient requires, and that's it. The order flows one way—physician to hospital.

In our bottleneck model (Chapter 9), the bed count is the bottleneck and the physician is the sole upstream stage. Recall the role of the upstream stages: The sole purpose of the stage(s) of production upstream of the bottleneck is to keep the bottleneck busy generating revenue.

Okay, but surely the bottleneck is only going to be generating revenue if the patient is bringing revenue and if the bottleneck service matches up with the patient's need.

In the simple MRI center example in Chapter 4, we took pains to reduce the number of stages upstream of the bottleneck to reduce

Figure 12.1. Basic Admission Order

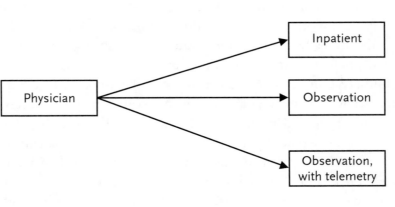

Going Lean: Busting Barriers to Patient Flow

the variability and the risk that the bottleneck—the MRI machine, in that case—would run out of work. Here, we go in the opposite direction. We add an upstream stage to protect the bottleneck from inappropriate consumption of bottleneck capacity. So, let's introduce a stage just before the bottleneck and give it a name. Let's call it the patient-flow control desk (see Figure 12.2).

In the figure, the little arrow is shown pointing in both directions to convey the notion that a dialog takes place. It's not just one way now. After clearing administrative matters, the doctor and the desk agent work quickly through a set of standard-of-care criteria to reach a common understanding on where the patient should go within the hospital. Using national criteria makes this an impartial screen, not an argument over whose professional judgment should prevail.

There are two prominent sets of care criteria. Any general hospital could establish its own, although it generally simplifies matters to use one of the national sets, and because insurance companies and government agencies use the same ones.

1. Milliman Care Guidelines (2006) produces annually updated, evidence-based clinical guidelines that cover the continuum of care, including ambulatory care, inpatient and surgical care, general recovery care, recovery facility care, home care, and chronic care.
2. McKesson (2006) InterQual solutions are clinical decision support to deliver evidence that works in managed care organizations, hospitals, and outpatient settings.

Figure 12.2. Admission Order with Flow Control

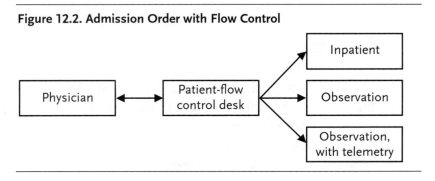

The dialog goes something like this:

Doctor: I wish to order the admission of John Doe.
Desk agent: Thank you. Let me run through the checklist.
Doctor: [Sighs.]
Desk agent: Here we go [pulls out the checklist].

Admissions Checklist Dialog			
Question	**Inpatient**	**Observation**	**Deny**
1. Is the patient self-pay?			
2. Is Mr. Doe on the do-not-admit list?			
3. Is Mr. Doe on the inpatient-only list?			
4. Observe/inpatient checklist, ask about the McKesson InterQual list.			
5. Does Mr. Doe require any special equipment?			
6. We will admit Mr. Doe if you write your admission order accordingly. Thank you.			

All this would be subject to appeal by the doctor to the next highest administrative level and would require support from senior management if the appeal is to do any good. Remember when the patient on the stretcher was thought to be the governor (Chapter 1)? We said then that the system can accommodate one super-priority patient but not a throng of super-priority patients. Every physician is apt to think that the patient at hand deserves special, super-priority consideration. Even if that were so for this particular patient, the system as a whole won't work that way. It can't. The hospital does not have infinite capacity. There is a bottleneck.

If there were only one patient, as in our case of Mr. Doe, this would all be very simple. In reality, there are lots of doctors and lots of patients, so there are lots of reasons to have a basic patient-flow control desk to provide discipline to the process.

FLOW-CONTROLLED ADMISSIONS

Let's look at the more general case. In Figure 12.3 we have several inflows of patients, each with a doctor writing an admission order. The arrows all point to the right because each doctor is writing an order unilaterally.

With the patient-flow control desk inserted (see Figure 12.4), this becomes a two-stage process, with a dialog between the doctors

Figure 12.3. General Admission

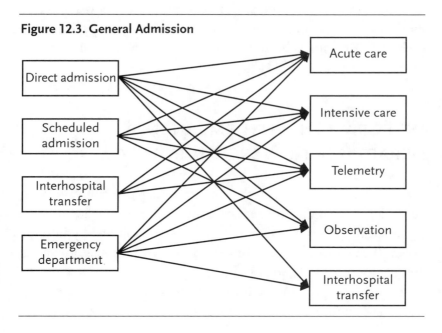

Figure 12.4. Admission with Flow Control

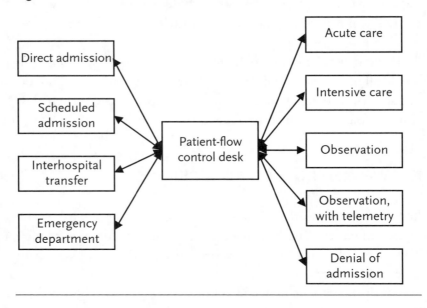

and the control desk. The two-headed arrows mean dialog. This model can be taken to a finer structure to deal with specialization such as burn units. The script for the dialog here is the same as described earlier.

INTEGRATION WITH EMERGENCY DEPARTMENT DIVERSION POLICY

If the number of patients in the emergency department waiting for admission exceeds the number established by hospital policy, or if the projected holdup time exceeds the number established by hospital policy, then patients can be transferred to other hospitals, incoming ambulances can be diverted to other hospitals, or both.

Senior management needs to set those policy limits on holdup count and holdup time, and senior management needs to assign the authority to transfer and the authority to divert either to emergency department management or to the patient-flow control desk. The assignment of authority needs to be unambiguous.

Note

1. A statistical number of CT scans were figured into the prospective, fixed-fee payment formula for inpatients, so no additional payment is warranted.

References

McKesson. 2006. InterQual Decision Support. [Online information; retrieved 9/12/06.] www.mckesson.com/en_us/McKesson.com/ For+Healthcare+Providers/Surgery+Centers/Clinical+Decision+Support/ InterQual+Decision+Support+for+Providers.html.

Milliman Care Guidelines. 2006. [Online information; retrieved 9/12/06.] www.careguidelines.com.

CHAPTER 13

Surgery

Some hospitals find that the first surgery in the morning never starts on time. Whether this is a universal issue or not, it's an interesting one. Late-starts bog down the whole day. Minutes lost in the morning cannot be recaptured during the day—they're just gone. What to do?

COPING WITH VARIABILITY BY DESIGN

If it were possible to prepare the operating room for both Surgeon A's case and for Surgeon B's case, then the first surgeon through the door would get the operating room and the other one can wait. Or, if it were possible to switch the room over instantaneously, the first surgeon through the door would get the operating room. Rapid switchover is desirable on its own because it maximizes the portion of the day that can be productive. The more rapid the switchover, the more that first-in, first-out rule can be applied to surgeons. Or, if Surgeon A's patient or nurse is delayed, or anything else comes along, it's good if the room can be switched over rapidly.

Production of the surgery department depends, in part, on how well the system is designed to cope with variability, which is a recurring theme of this book, as the reader will have noticed by now. Some variability can be controlled; some cannot. Take steps to control those that can be controlled, and take steps to tolerate those that cannot be controlled.

For instance, if three operating rooms are equipped identically, then a delay in one of them will not hold production up very much because the next patient on the roster can go to the next available room. If each room is specialized, then the system as a whole is less able to respond to upsets and delays. Identical operating rooms make the whole day's schedule much more predictable, to the benefit of all parties, because the only parameter that needs to be known to do the forecasting is the average completion time. Exceptions average out. So, it would be worthwhile to determine what it would take, if anything, to make some operating rooms identical and equally suitable for the bulk of surgical cases. Or the same, by subsets of operating rooms and patients.

Identical means identical—same size, same orientation, same windows, same doors, same switch positions, same plumbing, same lighting, same supply carts, same everything. Left-hand/right-hand configurations are bad. Rooms that are almost the same but not quite are bad, too. Go for identical; that applies to the first surgeries of the day, too. If most cases are ready to go on time, then the impact of one or two late-starts averages out. Late-starts don't help, but they don't hurt as much if subsets of the operating rooms are equipped identically.

COPING WITH VARIABILITY BY STRATEGY

There are two other known solutions to getting the first surgery of the morning to launch on time. One is to sort things around so that surgeons who like to start early get the early bookings. This can be done by letting surgeons bid or self-nominate for the early times. Another is to post a tracking chart of on-time launches. For best results, the tracking chart should just show the performance of the aggregate of all surgeons. The chart might track minutes lost to late-starts per day.

Post the chart in a conspicuous place, and let nature take its course. Two different chief medical officers have remarked to us that doctors are so competitive by nature that if score is being kept, they want to win. It doesn't matter what the game is. If the game is minutes not lost, doctors want to win.

PLANNING AND PREPARING FOR UPSETS

One of the uncontrollable sources of variability is the true condition of the patient. The surgical system does best if it can cope with a wide range of variability. Coping includes planning for a wide range of upsets that might happen during the surgery, including poor or inadequate training, shortage of supplies on hand, and pre-planned courses of action.

Training needs to include the whole surgical team and a wide range of possible upsets. That's done with computerized manikins these days (see Chapter 15). Taking the whole team, including the bench players, to be trained as a team seems to provide the best results.

> Air Force pilots have a checklist to follow before bailing out, even if the plane is on fire.

The hospital should have standard protocols for each type of surgery. These are usually provided by national standards groups within each specialty. The standard should be documented in a script and a flowchart, with a checklist designed to track events. For each credible upset, the revised course of action should be laid out in the same way, with a script, a flowchart, and a checklist. These not only provide the bases for training, but they also serve as a basis for keeping track of things as directions change.

Dr. Atul Gawande (2005), noted lecturer on patient safety and writer for the *New Yorker* on medical matters, says that leaving a sponge behind is de facto evidence of malpractice. Yet, it is very rare that a sponge is left behind in an ordinary surgery, where the sponges are counted as many as eight times. Rather, sponges and implements get left behind when the planned course of the surgery could not be followed for unexpected reasons or if the surgery took an unexpected turn. Dr. Gawande cites one case where two eight-inch clamps were left behind. One was found the same day by x-ray. The other was not found until two years later. Dr. Gawande looked into the hospital records and found 54 parallel cases with no clamps left behind. What happened in that particular case?

Sponges are left behind once in about 15,000 cases. That sounds pretty good, but with at least 1 million surgical procedures per month in the United States, that statistic means hundreds of compromised patients per year. About two-thirds of such events cause serious complications for the patient. Sponge errors are ten times more likely in emergency surgery. Sponge errors are four times more likely when the diagnosis was wrong, which is to say when the surgeon expected to see A and found B instead, necessitating a midstream change in the procedure.

All the more reason to train the whole team for upsets, prepare for upsets, document that preparation, and have checklists ready to use.

SPECIALIZATION

Specialization not only brings special knowledge to the patient but also the operational benefit of habit and repetition. Specialization in advanced medical practice, such as liver transplant, is to be expected. Specialization in rather ordinary matters, such as hernia repair, has been shown to be beneficial to the patient, not only because the surgery goes faster and is less likely to need redoing but also because the surgeon will more readily recognize off-normal conditions and cope with exceptions. Shouldice Hernia Center in Toronto, Canada, does only hernia surgeries (see www.shouldice.com). Ten surgeons do 7,500 procedures a year. By specializing, the group has had the opportunity to develop new procedures that appear to have advanced the state of the art, which is perhaps to be expected.

TECHNOLOGY FOR UPSET PRECLUSION

There are high expectations in the general public that technology is going to solve all medical problems. It is good to be hopeful. It is prudent to be cautious. In the language of this book, the public is hopeful that technology will provide a breakthrough.

Take the matter of marking the site for surgery. That's certainly a good idea. There are even computer chips specifically designed and FDA approved for subcutaneous marking of the site and/or paste-on marking on the site (see www.verichipcorp. com). That takes care of finding the site when the patient is draped for surgery, but how does the surgeon know that the chip was implanted at the proper site?

> There are surgical sponges with RFID chips (Roebuck 2004).

It is customary now to have the patient mark the site or to confirm that the correct side of the body is being marked. Is the patient a sufficient or competent authority? There is a known case where the patient was, in fact, himself a surgeon who participated in the marking before being anesthetized but still marked the wrong side of his own body (Barach 2006). How can technology help that? There are also known cases where the standard method of marking was done, with arrows drawn with full knowledge of the patient, but the surgeon still amputated the wrong toe. This one may take more than technology.

Where technology seems to work well in surgery is by providing productivity to the surgeon and to others on the surgical team—that is, technology helping the surgeon do the task, but not replacing the surgeon. This includes remote surgery, with machines far away being controlled by the movements of the surgeon nearby. This includes robotic surgical machines that prepare bone surfaces in hip surgery, doing what the surgeon would do and adding a measure of precision. In such technology, the surgeon can grasp what the machine is doing while the machine has a limited range of functionality and therefore introduces only a limited range of risk.

TRANSFER AND PATIENT FLOW

Many patients go from surgery to an inpatient bed. Therefore, surgery is upstream of the bottleneck—the inpatient bed count. Because patients are also flowing in from other upstream sources, such as the emergency department, it is disruptive to the system if the surgery patients are all transferred as a batch. It's better to transfer them one at a time. This is facilitated by a policy saying that the patient is ready for transfer when the patient has, for instance, vital signs within a planned range. When the patient is medically ready, then start the transfer process. This keeps the surgical nurses paying an extra modicum of attention to the progress of the patient, and it tends to smooth out the transfers over time.

It also helps to keep the patient flow-control desk currently informed on the number of patients to be transferred and when and what special requirements are going to be needed so that the department getting the patient will have a bed reserved and any special equipment on hand. There is even a school of thought on IV lines. That school of thought says that it is better to keep IV lines from getting snarled before the patient is moved than to unsnarl the IV lines later.

References

Barach, P. 2006. Lecture at the American Society for Quality, Milwaukee, Wisconsin, July.

Gawande, A. 2005. Lecture at the Carnegie Music Hall, Pittsburgh, Pennsylvania, February.

Roebuck, K. 2004. "Surgical Tracking Device Soaks Up Top Honors." *Pittsburgh Tribune Review* (March 30).

Western Reserve Care System[1] in Youngstown, Ohio, has two progressive ICUs, one of which is dedicated to postsurgery patients. Many patients flow to this ICU and then to a bed in a progressive care unit. As with all ICUs, keeping patients longer than necessary is a self-imposed burden that does nothing for the patient. A barrier to patient flow.

The decision to release the patient is made by the physician, perhaps prompted by ICU nurses, based on the vital signs presented by the patient and consistent with postsurgery expectations.

GETTING IT TO HAPPEN

Clear lines of authority, clear professional responsibilities, and clear medical indicia are necessary, and they are present. They are not quite enough. It's necessary for the authorized doctor to pull the trigger to release the patient.

That seems to be simple enough, and yet the simplest things don't do themselves.

LOCAL OPTIMIZATION

The responsible ICU nurse is patient-care oriented and task oriented by natural proclivity and professional training. Those are personal and tangible qualities. Thinking about a release is at least one stage more abstract, requiring longitudinal rather than task-now thinking for at least a moment. The nurse naturally optimizes in favor of caring for the patient rather than moving the patient along. While patient care certainly trumps patient flow, once the patient is sufficiently recovered from surgery to be suitable for care in a regular hospital department, there is no further patient-care benefit to keeping that patient in the surgery ICU.

A SELF-COMMUNICATION AID

In every shift for every patient, an orange form (see Figure 13.1) is inserted on top of all the other forms on the patient's clipboard. At the very top, there is one question similar to "Why is this patient still here?"

Lines follow this question, allowing a quick check-off for likely medical reasons, but those don't really matter. What really matters is that the nurse has to think for a moment and ask, why is this patient still here? This self-communication aid works better than having the supervisor pose the same question. Self-communication is more likely to get a reasoned answer, and it doesn't take up the supervisor's time.

The form itself, filled out, becomes part of the record and documents the professional view held by the responsible nurse at that time. That's worthwhile, but it is secondary to the value of self-communication.

Note

1. One of the book's coauthors, Amy Smith, is director of case management at this healthcare system.

Figure 13.1. Orange Form

MICU Patient Daily Goals

What is being done for this patient that cannot be done in a lower level of care?	Technology, i.e., ventilator Intensive monitoring, i.e., VS q 1h-2h Intensive intervention, i.e., titrate drips
Is patient ready for transfer?	YES NO

<table>
<tr><td rowspan="4">Daily Review</td><td>Code Status:</td><td colspan="2">Daily Labs Review:</td></tr>
<tr><td colspan="3">Central Line Management: Triple/Quad PA Vascath PICC
Is/Are Lines Necessary?</td></tr>
<tr><td>Tests/Procedures</td><td colspan="2">Glasgow < 5/vented with neuro insult?
CALL LIFEBANC</td></tr>
</table>

<table>
<tr><th colspan="2">Plan/Goal to be Achieved</th><th>RN 7a–7p Reviewed (initial)</th><th>RN 7p–7a Reviewed (initial)</th></tr>
<tr><td rowspan="6">Shift Review, General</td><td>Family communications and psychological social services needed</td><td></td><td></td></tr>
<tr><td>Inter-service communications and pending consultations</td><td></td><td></td></tr>
<tr><td>Pain management</td><td></td><td></td></tr>
<tr><td>Sedation management</td><td></td><td></td></tr>
<tr><td>Infection isolation, e.g., cultures, antibiotics, levels</td><td></td><td></td></tr>
<tr><td>Medications, e.g., change meds, check levels, renal adjustment</td><td></td><td></td></tr>
</table>

Continued...

Plan/Goal to be Achieved			RN 7a–7p Reviewed (initial)	RN 7p–7a Reviewed (initial)
Shift Review, Systems	Neurologic, e.g., seizures, LOC, speech evaluation			
	Cardiovascular, e.g., volume, rhythm, hemodynamics, DVT			
	Respiratory, e.g., ventilator, SaO$_2$, weaning?			
	Endocrine, blood sugar <110 insulin gtt, conversion to subq tx			
	Hematologic, e.g., transfusions, platelet count			
	Renal, e.g., dialysis, urine output			
	GI/nutrition, HOB 30 degrees, PUD, e.g., passing stool, flatus, nutrition			
	Mobility/skin/extremities activity, PT, OT, e.g., Decub prevention ROM			

Signature:

Physician: _____ Clinical Pharmacist: _____

7a–7p Nurse: _____ 7p–7a Nurse: _____

Respiratory Therapist: _____ Dietitian:_____

Other: _____ Other: _____

Source: Recreated with permission from Western Reserve Care System, Youngstown, Ohio.

CHAPTER 14

Inpatient Care

This is the bottleneck. Execution is everything.

BACKGROUND

The role of the hospital is to care for patients. The business of the hospital is to care for patients and to get paid for doing so. Getting paid requires getting the paperwork right.

Medicare will now condition payments to hospitals, not only on diagnosis but also on severity of the patient's condition. Medicare will base its payment to the hospital on the medical record written by the attending physician. Therefore, the hospital has a paramount need to get the physician to write up the patient's record thoroughly, enumerating all the complicating factors exhibited by the patient.

The hospital has always depended on the cooperation of the physician in essential matters—one obvious one being the fact that the hospital has no basis for billing the payer until the physician signs the physician's portion of the patient's record. While this new Medicare policy makes more work for the hospital and for the physician, it is only fair to say that Medicare took this new step in response to every hospital saying, "Our patients have more complications than the average." Hospitals now have the opportunity to prove this to be so and to be paid accordingly. Now, in addition to executing well on patient care, hospitals need to execute well on patient care documentation. Hospitals need to staff and to operate accordingly.

HOSPITALIST SPECIALIZATION

A recent development in physician specialization is the hospitalist. Hospitalists specialize in the role of attending physician, working within the hospital, with patients being handed over to the hospitalist after the admission order is written by the admitting physician.

As with any medical specialization, the expectation is that physicians who specialize in attending will, through repetition and hands-on learning, become more skilled in this phase of medical practice than will other doctors who deal with a wider range of activities. This development is supported by family doctors who make other use of their time, receive fewer phone calls in the middle of the night, and benefit from reduced malpractice premium rates.

For the hospital, dealing with a modest number of hospitalists rather than with hundreds of other doctors goes in the direction of easier communications and better consistency of execution. Hospitalists are often members of the National Association of Inpatient Physicians.

The Hospital–Hospitalist Relationship

The Medicare policy changes mentioned earlier make it all the more important that the hospital have a suitable relationship with the hospitalist. If the hospitalist is an employee of the hospital or contracts directly with the hospital, then the relationship can be written into a contract stipulating actions to be taken. For instance, the hospitalist is to conform to the hospital's standard protocols and records policies, and the physician's portion of the patient's record is to be signed at the time the discharge order is written.

CASE MANAGEMENT

Bedside nurses are task oriented, planning and executing a list of tasks for each patient in their charge that day. Case managers, who are most commonly nurses themselves, take the longitudinal view of each patient's care from admission (or, better yet, preadmission) through inpatient care through discharge (or postdischarge).

The case manager identifies each patient's payer sources upon admission, communicates with payers, and secures payer authorizations. The case manager deals with noncoverage notices and appeals. The case manager recommends resources consistent with the patient's need and tracks the patient's progress. The case manager looks for barriers affecting any patient—in particular, barriers that are recurring or systematic. Clearing away such barriers is in everybody's interest. Case managers monitor providers' utilization of resources for appropriateness and timeliness, and they intervene as needed to ensure that essential services are delivered at the most appropriate level of care. Case managers ensure that the patient's care plan is consistent with hospital standards, that the care plan is being carried out, and that all the mandatory records are completed concomitantly.

> Case managers have a longitudinal rather than a task view of the patient.

The origin of case management was in the realization that there are sociological aspects of patient care that reach beyond the hospital. That belief continues and is reflected in the presence of social workers in most case management departments. Case management departments have the following responsibilities.

Clinical Care Coordination

Start by confirming that the physician's order conforms to the hospital's standard protocol. If not, resolve the situation with the attending physician. In cases where the treatment will very likely run a predictable course, no further attention from the case manager is likely to be needed. In cases where the course of events cannot be predicted with high confidence at admission, then continuing attention from the case manager is likely to be necessary. For example, a patient coming in for a scheduled laparoscopic gallbladder removal probably will not need ongoing case management, while a patient coming in for a colon resection probably will.

In instances where the case manager has continuing involvement, the case manager's interest is to confirm that the hospital's standard protocols are being applied and that hospital resources are being provided. Case managers often participate in conferences with the patient's family. Case managers document interventions and referrals in the case manager's progress notes.

Psychosocial Care Coordination

Patients who have complicating factors beyond their medical condition need additional care or help. The case manager coordinates with specialists and social workers, as may be appropriate, to support the patient's need. Case managers document screening results, referrals, and interventions in the case manager's progress notes.

Clinical Documentation Management

Case managers track clinical documentation. This is a heightened responsibility under the new Medicare regime because payment to the hospital by Medicare depends on the severity of the patient's condition, as described in the physician's portion of the patient record. Medicare has its own lexicon, and for the hospital to be paid appropriately, the hospital has to persuade the physician to use the Medicare lexicon.

One well-known example is the total hip replacement, in which a substantial loss of blood during the operation is normal. The next day, the patient will very likely be anemic. Because this is the expected course of events, the surgeon is not likely to remark upon it in the physician's record. Medicare recognizes blood-loss anemia as a complication meriting additional payment. So, it is in the hospital's interest to ask the surgeon to note this anemia in the record so that the true state of the patient is captured in the documentation.

The orthopedic surgeon, while interested to see the hospital receive appropriate payment, may not want the record to imply that the patient has had more than normal blood loss, which might be taken as a reflection on the surgeon's competence. The hospital and its orthopedic surgeons need to come to a common understanding of how to document this matter. Once an agreement has been reached, the case manager reviews the patient's records to confirm that policy is being followed and, where not, to request that the physician make conforming entries in the record.

This is but one example. Our point is that the hospital needs documentation standards as well as protocol standards and that tracking conformance to documentation standards is an important business function that the hospital needs to perform. The hospital is dependent on doctors' cooperation. The case manager, as documentation manager, seeks to have timely signatures on all records as well.

Utilization Management and Payer Coordination

Case managers apply clinical criteria to the medical record to determine the medical necessity for

> Utilization management is not meant to keep the facility full; it is meant to accelerate patient flow.

a given level of care. In addition, they communicate these criteria to the patient's insurance company, if applicable, to secure authorization for payment. The case manager may also coordinate the appeals process should payment authorization be denied.

Discharge Planning

Case managers begin discharge planning upon admission, but preferably before admission. Where's the patient going to go, and how is the patient going to get there? When? Who's going to be on hand when the patient gets there? Only one of these is under any measure of hospital control—the when—and even that one requires a doctor's order. The others require the cooperation of outside parties.

Communicating with these outside parties is key. One important party is the patient. It is helpful to inform the patient, "you will be ready to go home when you can walk 100 feet on your own, or when you can change your own colostomy bag." That's better than telling the patient "five days," because it gets the patient directly involved in getting ready to go home. Telling the patient's family the same thing goes in the right direction, as does giving the family periodic reports on the patient's progress toward qualifying for discharge.

Preadmission Coordination

Hospital stays nowadays are so short, and getting shorter, that discharge planning needs to happen before admission for as many nonurgent patients as possible. It is becoming common to bring patients to a briefing several days before elective surgery to explain to them and their family what to expect upon arrival, what to expect after surgery, what to expect each day thereafter, and what the medium and long-term effects will be. It is important that discharge planning be included in that briefing. Where there is some prospect that the patient may need to be transferred to a rehabilitation center upon discharge, and particularly when it cannot be known with certainty whether that transfer will be required or not, this needs to be covered in the preadmission briefing.

This preadmission activity is worthwhile for all admissions. Financial requirements, insurance conditions, copays, and so on all need to be covered in the preadmission sessions for the peace of mind of the patient and the patient's family. For scheduled admissions, this is straightforward. The same would be desirable for non-scheduled admissions as well. In this case, of course, the patient is not knowable per se, but there are things that can be done. For instance, nursing home residents in the service area are likely candidates for eventual hospital care. So are sports teams, motorcycle clubs, persons doing physical or hazardous work, and affiliation groups such as people with diabetes and disabled veterans. The hospital can reach out to these populations periodically to work out some of the essentials, including

1. Who is going to identify the patient? The van driver?
2. Who has family telephone numbers?
3. Who has power of attorney?
4. Is there a family physician of record?
5. Who is the point of contact at the hospital?

Having this information in hand can only help the patient and the hospital alike.

These days, when most people are Internet savvy, it is quite possible to encourage self-declaration of such information on a suitable website that provides privacy assurance. Some third-party websites encourage the user to enter his medical history. That might be helpful, although it introduces lots of questions. Suppose the patient states on an online form: "no allergy to penicillin." How much weight should that be given?

Postdischarge Coordination

The patient's discharge order very likely includes postdischarge orders for medicine, diet, exercise, follow-up doctor appointments, follow-up lab exams, and perhaps visiting nurse home visits. It is in the hospital's interest that patients adhere to these instructions, both because it is in the patient's favor and because the hospital may have difficulty getting reimbursed if the patient is readmitted soon after discharge. This starts with making sure the postdischarge instructions are included in the discharge order.

Documentation Management

If visiting nurse service is ordered, it is to be expected that the visiting nurse will make sure the patient and supporting family members understand the doctor's instructions. If no visiting nurse service is ordered, it is in the hospital's interest to make follow-up phone calls for this purpose.

One postdischarge activity that has been found to be effective is to invite kindred patients to attend group meetings with a nurse who goes over the progress to be expected, reminds patients to follow their instructions, and answers questions. Patients are encouraged to report any change in weight or other factors that might indicate a change in condition. It seems that patients enjoy and benefit from this social interaction with other patients. While there is always a risk that such sessions encourage hypochondria, the general run of experience is that patients stay interested in their own recovery, pay more attention to their instructions, and want to attend the next meeting. For some groups, such as cancer patients undergoing therapy, these sessions have been found to evolve as mutual-support meetings, with patients counseling each other and sharing their own experiences. These patients are not only interested in their own progress, they are also interested in the progress of their newfound friends.

Recently, insurance companies and other interested parties have sponsored coaching by telephone. A coach telephones a list of patients—adult diabetics are commonly targeted—to ask questions. What did you eat yesterday? What medicine did you take yesterday? What did you weigh this morning? What alcohol did you drink yesterday? Are you smoking? And so on. The questions are specific to the patient's known condition and recently supplied information. This sounds a lot like nagging, which has not had too much of a track record as a way of sustaining preferred patterns of behavior these past 6,000 years.

A similar, but non-nagging, method has been tried by the Veterans Administration, which provides a secure web page and asks patients to self-report each day. This seems to do the trick. A medical professional reviews the information to flag exceptions. Readmissions are down, and upsets are caught earlier. Call it self-nagging.

It is in the hospital's interest to see that these things get done. If they are being done by others, fine. If not, the hospital should consider doing these things directly or steering patients with chronic conditions to a suitable source of support.

INPATIENT BARRIERS TO PATIENT FLOW

Because the point is to take care of patients, and because observation is being pushed in this book as an important place to start, how can the flow of patients be observed?

To get started, it's instructive to follow one patient all the way through the care process. Take lots of notes. Then, follow another one, and then a few more, one at a time. This takes a little patience, because we are all geared to pounce on problems and solve them. It's better, though, to get enough patient-flow histories so that useful generalizations can be made and the system can be improved in a managed way. That will be better than lots of Band-Aids to fix specific problems.

Conemaugh Memorial Medical Center in Johnstown, Pennsylvania, worked with the Joint Commission to follow a few individual patients all the way through the system; these were named "tracer patients" (PRHI 2004). The team selected a patient at random, one who happened to have come in with chest pains leading to a cardiac catheterization exam. As it happens, no blockages were found, and the patient was due to be released when the team visited the patient's bedside. The patient gave positive answers to all questions and was very happy with the service. With this perfect patient, perfect service, and perfect outcome, the team thought that maybe this one was too easy, nothing would be learned. Even so, to follow through on its plan, the team then interviewed the nurse caring for this patient. Lots of questions were asked, including what-if questions. Open discussion. Notes taken.

Then the team visited the cardiac catheterization lab and interviewed the nurse in charge. What might be fixed here? "It takes hours to get meds," was the answer. Then the team walked all the way through the system to touch on every unit involved in any way with this patient. Lab. Wheelchair inventory. Billing. When all the notes were consolidated, the team decided that while the patient went home happy, they had found 27 deficiencies in the system. Those deficiencies, in this case, did not prevent the patient from getting good care, but they still needed attention. Action items were written for some; studies were ordered for others.

Conemaugh Memorial's senior management decided to make a once-a-week follow of a "tracer patient" a permanent feature. (It would be interesting to learn how often the same problem pops back up. Do-it fixes, rather than systematic fixes, tend to make problems pop back up in the same place or in the next department. The barrier seems to move rather than go away. If they pop up a second time, look deeper for a systematic change.) Incidentally, this exercise led the team to reduce the waiting time for a first chemotherapy dose from 6 hours (average for 30 patients) to 2.5 hours and currently to 30 minutes. That's a nice improvement in patient flow.

CONVERGENCE OF INTERESTS

Let's consider a few common cases where the parties' interests are not quite converged in the direction of maximum patient flow.

Five-Day Week, Seven-Day Demand

The hospital runs seven days a week because the demand on the hospital runs seven days a week. Emergency and obstetrics departments plan and staff accordingly. Physicians in these specialties either work all seven days themselves or find ways, in small groups, to cover weekends, vacations, and holidays. In these cases, the demand for physician services as well as hospital services declares itself. Physicians respond; the hospital responds. No barrier. Those are easy.

Other matters take more management attention. For example, a patient appears on a Friday with chest discomfort, and a cardiac catheterization is ordered. The patient is stable. Not an emergency. When does the patient get the catheterization? Saturday? Sunday? Monday? If Monday is a holiday, then Tuesday? Looks like a barrier to patient flow. Does it matter?

Yes. And not just because the bed is not generating additional revenue and some incremental costs for food and housekeeping are being borne. Two-thirds of "preventable" hospital deaths appear to be from nosocomial infection. Every day the patient is in the hospital is another day when contagion lurks. The patient may well receive visitors, and visitors bring in germs. The patient knows, and so does the patient's family, that the exam is being put off for the convenience of somebody other than the patient. The patient's frustration, waiting for the exam, may well be exacerbated by other minor waits. Such patients are the very ones who decide not to wait for someone to help them get to the toilet and who would get out of bed on their own and take a tumble. So, it is in everybody's interest, except perhaps the cardiologist's, to give the catheterization exam promptly, to remove this barrier to patient flow.

What to do? Get weekend coverage. How? Negotiate with cardiologist groups to get weekend and holiday coverage. If the cardiologists are not employees, then there is not much that hospital management can do unilaterally. Negotiations are required. While at first blush the cardiologists hold all the cards, given that they are the only ones who are going to be doing the catheterizations, in this case the hospital has the patient. The admission was very likely ordered by the patient's family doctor, who then ordered the cardiac examination. So hospital management has a few cards to play, too. Negotiate to remove this barrier.

Licensed Scope of Practice

Under law and regulations, certain healthcare professionals are licensed to do things that others are not. These licensed scopes of practice are often challenged at the fringe. Often the case in point is what doctor-like actions a nurse practitioner is allowed to do. Or when a pharmacist must be physically present in a drug store.

Because these are matters of law and regulation, they are open to challenge through the agency review and legislative processes. They are also open to close scrutiny to determine whether an item is written into present regulations or is simply a matter of tradition. Those who hold licensed privileges are apt to use that license to the holder's advantage. It is only natural, and it is in the holder's pecuniary interest, to protect the licensed exclusivity. Licensed exclusivity encourages local optimization, in favor of the license holder and not in favor of good patient flow. Barriers. Good patient flow is in the patient's favor. Here's an example.

A patient is brought in with apparent stroke. Standard practice mandates an examination of the patient's ability to swallow before the patient is given anything by mouth. That's prudent, and if the exam is done promptly, then everything is fine. Swallow exams are done by speech pathologists. If there are speech pathologists on hand and standing by, that's fine. If there are speech pathologists with other things to do that delay doing the swallow exam, then the patient is discomfited and patient flow is arrested. Barrier.

Is the swallow exam, under license, to be done only by speech pathologists? It turns out that there is no such exclusive right (but it should be verified in each state). Nurses can be trained to do the swallow exam and are not barred from doing it. This eliminates a barrier. Eliminating barriers is the whole idea.

Interfacing Departments

Many patients move from one department to another, perhaps to a third, in the course of their treatment. Each department has its own operational and professional interests in the progress of the patient. The professional interests of each department do not clash with one another, but neither do they necessarily line up in a way that gives best patient flow.

Surgery patients are kept in the surgery department until they are stable. Surgery patients are, not infrequently, kept beyond the stable point and then transferred all at once (or so it seems to the next department). Transferring all at once leads to a line of stretchers in hallways, which is not in the patient's favor. It may certainly be argued that keeping that patient for an extra hour or so in the surgery department is in the patient's favor, just in case something develops.

However, that argument has to have an end to it at some time, or else all patients would stay in the surgery department until they are ready to go home. There is a medical basis for the standard protocol, including the determination of when a patient is ready for transfer. If the protocol needs to be changed, fine. Until then, follow it.

Here is an opportunity to apply self-benchmarking. The benchmark is, transfer when patient is stable. This is a self-benchmark because the standard—the benchmark—arises from local information. All the information needed is already in hand; it is qualified for use because it is part of the standard protocol, and the only thing required is to do it. Do it every time. There are just three steps to take:

1. Establish the benchmark.
2. Tell people what is now expected.
3. Make conformance visible.

Here, the benchmark is already established, and telling people what is now expected requires only one announcement at a group meeting. It is unlikely that any resistance will be mounted beyond the usual deep sighs brought on by any management directive. But that's not quite enough. Left to themselves, things will revert back to the prior practice. Something needs to be done to encourage conformance to the new policy, something that does not require clerks and clipboards.

What always works is to post a bar chart on the departmental bulletin board showing, perhaps monthly, a measure of conformance. In this case, a suitable measure might be the fraction of calls for transfer made within 15 minutes of the patient attaining stability. This will rise to approach 100 percent and will stay there because it is the nature of human beings to prefer a good score to a less-than-good score. The opposite might be posted—the fraction not conforming—with the intent that this number go in the direction of zero over time. That's rather negative in tone, don't you think? Positive-going scores are to be preferred.

Making such a tracking chart is not an undue burden on the departmental clerk; it is easy to understand, and it gives everybody something to feel good about each time the chart is updated on the bulletin board. Encouraging self-management is necessary when dealing with professionals, who don't like to be told what to do. Professionals do like to manage their own activities, which is fine, accompanied by a little guidance.

SUPPLY LINES

Hospital purchasing departments, left to themselves, assess their own performance by such measures as dollars saved by buying from the low-price supplier rather than the high-price supplier, inventory turns, supplier rationalization, local suppliers developed, and the like. These are all fine things indeed, and it would hardly be in the hospital's interest to buy from the high-price supplier, other things being equal. And while measures such as inventory turns show up directly on the balance sheet and have a direct bearing on cash balances, the overall goal is not to optimize inventory turns; it is to optimize overall system performance in favor of the patient.

Better measures might include

- hours of supply at point of use at maximum consumption rate,
- variability in time to replenish to point of use, and
- shelf-life expiry write-offs.

First of all, the focal point should be the point of use, not the storeroom. Second, the available resupply rate must be at least as great as the maximum consumption rate, or else supplies will eventually run out at the point of use. That means the supply chain needs to be highly predictable (low variability) and capable of responding to a peak in demand. Third, shelf-life expiry write-offs indicate that supplies are being ordered in too large a quantity. The purchasing instinct is to say that the consuming departments need to do a better job of forecasting need. This is not a likely course of events for most hospitals, where the variability comes with variable patients in variable numbers with variable conditions.

The supply line, as managed by the purchasing agents, needs to support both low consumption rates (to preclude shelf-life write-offs) and high consumption rates. To do so requires that the purchasing agents achieve a supply system with these characteristics:

1. Rapid and error-free consumption-rate information from point of use to the purchase agent and then to the supplier.
2. Rapid and reliable resupply from high-capacity suppliers.
3. Very low storeroom stocking levels.
4. Strategic backup planning in case of supply-line upset.

The storeroom stocking level is a measure of the imperfection of the supply line, which, no matter how good it is, cannot be expected to respond instantaneously. Promptly, yes. The more promptly the better, and the lower the storeroom stocking levels. Rapid resupply and low storeroom stocking levels mean that not much cash will be tied up in inventory and not much inventory will be written off at shelf-life expiry. It is much better to work on rapid resupply than to stock up inventory in the hopes of having enough to get to the next delivery date, particularly if that delivery date is not certain.

Note that buying low is not on the list. Buying low is far down on the priorities compared to not running out. Wal-Mart reinvented supply line management by applying information technology that was already available to everybody. Wal-Mart did not invent computers or barcodes or checkout scanners. Wal-Mart used these tools to get its supply line organized to have adequate quantities at the point of use (the store shelves), rapid resupply from vendors, and low storeroom (distribution center) inventory levels. While many vendors connected their own computer systems to the Wal-Mart computer system and carried the whole philosophy back through their own supply chains, reducing inventory at every point along the way, others did not. These others built their own warehouses across the street from Wal-Mart distribution centers.

There is a message here for local suppliers who want to qualify as suppliers to the hospital but who cannot have the production capability to respond to sudden peaks in demand the way a large supplier can. The message to the local supplier is, build your own warehouse and stock it to cover the highest conceivable consumption rate. Otherwise, you're not qualified.

Some hospitals are outsourcing all or part of supply management. That's fine, provided that the warranties of performance written into the outsourcing contract are based on "no outage at point of use no matter what the consumption rate may be."

Supplies and Patient Safety

Pittsburgh Regional Health Initiative (PRHI 2005) is a combined effort of many hospitals in western Pennsylvania to learn from the experiences of all. PRHI does a monthly newsletter. One article reported on patient-to-patient contagion experience, with a healthcare worker being the carrier. One patient was known to be a source of contagion and was kept in an isolation room. Healthcare workers were instructed to change gloves, gowns, and masks before and after entering that room. New gowns were stockpiled next to that door for convenience.

The supply of gowns by the door ran out. The healthcare worker decided to enter the room anyway, figuring that the patient needed her. That may or may not have been the right decision in those circumstances. It is clear, however, that running out of gowns was not the right thing.

Tucker Field Study

Professor Anita Tucker of Harvard Business School published an article in *California Management Review* entitled "Why Hospitals Don't Learn from Failures: Organizational and Psychological Dynamics that Inhibit System Change" (Tucker and Edmondson 2003). Professor Tucker sent business students to observe a number of hospitals to see what went wrong and to record those failures, great and small.

The psychological dynamic mentioned in the title is the (positive) psychology of nurses, who believe that the patient comes first and that their patient is *their* patient. If there are hurdles and encumbrances, get over them and take care of the patient. This positive is turned into a negative by Professor Tucker. A nurse was observed taking matters into her own hands when, at three o'clock in the morning, a bed needed to be changed and there were no fresh bed linens in the local supply cabinet. The nurse went to the next unit and grabbed some. That's good. No, that's bad, because the supply department can't look at the next requisition and adjust resupply quantities using standard business methods. Professor Tucker presents a solution in her article that appears to be another layer of administration. Our own informal survey finds that experienced nurses tend to hoard supplies so that they cannot run out. This may not work for bed linens, but it seems to be what happens with IV kits and even cardiac catheters. There are lots of reasons to wish this did not happen. Hoarding was not observed by Professor Tucker's students, but perhaps the study's experiment design did not have this in mind.

In sum, it appears to be the case that supply systems do not generate trust, and it appears to be the case that nurses take matters into their own hands as a consequence. If nurses do, others probably do as well. A workable solution is not likely to be another layer of management; it is more likely to be to clarify the role of the supply chain and to get global optimization, in favor of the patient, to include the supply chain.

Role of the Supply Chain

The purpose of the supply chain is to promote patient flow. An important part of that is to be trustworthy, providing a sufficient supply of everything all the time. The standard order-supply scheme is for a clerk to fill out a requisition, which goes to the supply center, which fills the order and delivers it to the order point.

Why not have the supply department itself fill out the order? That is to say, why not require the supply center to have an adequate inventory of everything at the point of use? Let the supply center assign someone to walk the floors and check the stock levels for bed linens, IV kits, and cardiac catheters. Handheld computers are routinely used to facilitate this in other industries, and not just in retailing.

> Pull systems minimize inventory and outages by creating simple small-lot reordering schemes. See Chapter 11 for a pull system that works.

While the reader will surely say that the supply clerk has no knowledge of medical need, the fact is that the ward clerk doesn't either. Both rely on historical consumption rates to predict future consumption rates, and the supply department is better equipped to deal with trends, patterns, statistical fluctuations, and anomalies than the ward clerk is; that's what supply management is all about these days. (This was Professor Tucker's point in the first place: scientific supply management requires valid input.) Make the supply department responsible for being trustworthy. Minimize inventory, develop suppliers, all those things, *after* taking care that there are no stockouts on items great and small at the point of use. Trust will follow, when it is earned. Hoards and caches will pass from style.

Develop appropriate measures and brag about attainment. This gives the purchasing department a visible, tangible, and valuable role in patient flow. That's good.

PATIENT INVOLVEMENT

People don't get well until they want to. Some people don't want to leave the hospital. Setting those aside, getting the patient involved in the patient's treatment and preparation to leave can only help.

Part of this is to work with the patient to make sure that the patient's next stop, whether home or a care facility, is planned and ready. Part of this is to get the patient thinking about discharge by such simple things as telling the patient, "Doctor says you can go home as soon as you can walk 100 steps." Part of this is to get the patient involved in staying well.

Here are some rules offered by the Central Manchester and Manchester Children's University Hospitals (2006):

1. Tell visitors to wash their hands before approaching your bed.
2. Tell visitors to stay home if they have the sniffles.
3. Tell visitors other than close family to stay home.
4. Tell doctors and nurses to wash their hands before approaching your bed.

5. Cooperate with the housekeeping staff who clean your room.
6. Keep visitors from sitting on your bed.

EMPLOYEE CONTRACTORS

Contractors are engaged by contract. The contract specifies scope, payment, and performance standards. Performance standards can include turnaround times.

As any provider moves to a patient-flow model, these contracts will need to carry the model change into performance-standard changes with specific attention paid to turnaround times. Each contract should call for standardized, trustworthy turnaround times for each deliverable. Cover all shifts. Contracts should call for external benchmarking, with renewals based on achieving parity with those external benchmarks.

Having done a few such contracts, senior management can then ask itself how to put those same performance standards before groups of employees to get the same performance characteristics. External benchmarking. Turnaround times that are standardized and trustworthy.

A contractor who fails to meet commitments is easy to deal with; get a different contractor. An employee group is harder to deal with because discharge and replacement are not likely to transpire. Still, the need to get to high achievement is real.

There is a school of thought that says it is never the employee who is coming up short, it is always the system (see www.deming.org). If the group is not achieving, improve the system. That might mean new tooling; it might mean renewed training; it might mean reassigning some people. Don't chastise the worker; fix the system. That's more management bother than changing contractors. It's also more satisfying when achievement is attained, and the improvement will abide.

See chapters 15 and 16 for inpatient care success stories.

References

Central Manchester and Manchester Children's University Hospitals. 2006. "Working Together to Beat the Bugs." [Online article; retrieved 9/12/06.] www.hpa.org.uk.

Pittsburgh Regional Health Initiative (PRHI). 2004. [Online newsletter, August; retrieved 9/12/06.] www.prhi.org.

———. 2005. "Contagion." [Online newsletter, October; retrieved 9/12/06.] www.prhi.org.

Tucker, A. L., and A. C. Edmondson. 2003. "Why Hospitals Don't Learn from Failures: Organizational and Psychological Dynamics that Inhibit System Change." *California Management Review* 45 (2): 55.

CHAPTER 15

External Benchmarking:
A Success Story

External benchmarking means recognizing clever work done
by others that can be adapted to your use.

BACKGROUND

The University of Pittsburgh Medical Center's Winter Institute for
Simulation, Education, and Research—UPMC WISER, for short—
uses computerized manikins to simulate real-life healthcare events and
develops the training programs that feature these manikins. Manikins
are remarkable these days, simulating everything from irregular
breathing to traumatic hemorrhage. More medical specialties are making use of them every year. The WISER success story, though, doesn't
start with manikins. This story starts with NASCAR pit crews.

The essence of external benchmarking is to recognize good ideas
when your gaze falls on them. Sometimes the external benchmark
is found in another hospital doing something that your hospital
does, only better. Sometimes it takes a little more imagination.

In virtually every hospital, patients who experience cardiac failure trigger a rapid-response team to rush to bedside to perform
resuscitation. The rapid-response team responds to a call using a

name such as "cardiac code" or just plain "code." Rapid action is in order. What does that have to do with NASCAR?

One WISER leader was watching a NASCAR race on television. The coverage always focuses on the pit crews, who pounce on the car when it comes into the pit, jack up the car, change the tires, fill the tank, give the driver liquid refreshment, clean the windshield, release the jacks, and get out of the way, all in a matter of seconds. What does that have to do with bedside cardiac resuscitation?

Here's where the simulation thought process comes in. Think of the NASCAR pit crew as simulating the cardiac rapid-response team. Okay, that's a bit of a stretch, but with a little imagination one can see that NASCAR organizes and manages the pit crew in a way that might help in thinking about how cardiac crisis teams might be quicker. Time is surely of the essence in both cases.

THE NASCAR MODEL

Here's how WISER boiled down the NASCAR pit crew model.

1. Every NASCAR pit crew member has an assigned task.
2. The next time, the pit crew member might well do a different task, but for this event, the crew member doing the right front tire is only doing the right front tire and nothing else.
3. Each crew member starts as soon as the car can be reached. Nobody waits for orders.
4. Nobody changes tasks in the middle.
5. Each crew member focuses on doing exactly the task assigned.

WISER considered this and decided that every position around the patient's bed can be assigned a position number and that the tasks for each position can be specified (DeVita et al. 2004).

Nurses and others can be trained in the duties of each position. Indeed, they can be trained to work at several different positions, but only one position is to be worked at a time.

WISER teams have eight members (see Figure 15.1):

Member	Assignment
1	Airway manager
2	Airway assistant
3	Bedside nurse
4	Crash cart nurse
5	Team leader
6	Chest compressions
7	Procedure MD
8	Recorder nurse

Figure 15.1. NASCAR Model for Crisis Teams

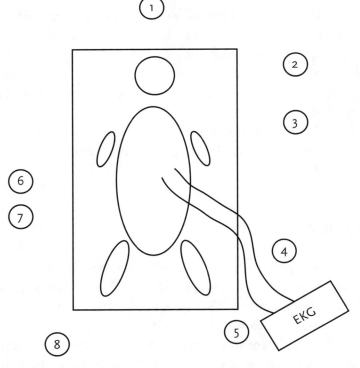

Source: Recreated with permission from UPMC WISER, Pittsburgh, Pennsylvania.

Position number 5 is the team leader. The role of the team leader is not to bark orders. Rather, it is to assess how the team is doing, analyze the data, direct treatment, and "triage to next care site." Note that treatment direction is in third rank, not first. Treatment is to be directed, or redirected, only after assessing the team and analyzing the data. The presumption is that the team starts things off in the right direction with no orders given and that each team member knows what to do at the position occupied.

Here's the WISER method for rapid response to a cardiac code:

1. Go to bedside.
2. Take an open position.
3. Go at it. Don't wait for orders or instructions.
4. Stay at that position, doing only the duties of that position.

Note that no adjustments to work assignments are made, even if a more qualified person arrives. So this is not a method for providing the best possible care; this is a method for providing prompt, qualified, and effective care. WISER's experience with this method is that the time from alert to care application is cut by half. That's pretty good.

WISER trains teams to operate in this way by using computerized manikin simulators. Training includes cardiac events, stroke, and opioid overdose.

REMARKS

In this book, we talk often of coping with variability. The time for each team member to get to bedside is certainly variable, falling beyond anyone's control. It's uncontrollable variability. Given that that variability is uncontrollable, the best thing to do is to desensitize the flow of the treatment to that variability. Telling the team to self-organize, spontaneously, on the basis of who gets there first is one way to do it.

Note

Management at WISER provided additional information in this chapter.

Reference

DeVita, M., J. Schaefer, T. Dongilli, H. Wang, and J. Lutz . 2004. "Improving Medical Crisis Team Performance Using a Computerized Patient Simulator." [Online article on UPMC WISER site; retrieved 5/28/07.] www.wiser.pitt.edu.

CHAPTER 16

Infection Reduction:
A Success Story

Precluding hospital-acquired infection is a good way to improve patient flow.

BACKGROUND

Hospitals use millions of catheters a year. Each event carries some potential for infection. Most serious infections arise with central-venous catheters, especially for ICU patients. About 15 million patient-days of central-venous catheterization occur annually in the United States, and bloodstream infections result in about 80,000 of these cases (CDC 2002). The Centers for Disease Control and Prevention (CDC) has been collecting data on such infections since the 1970s to provide information for the development of suitable methods of care and prevention. The CDC has issued guidelines. These guidelines include selection of the insertion site, hand hygiene, antiseptic cleansing of the site, and the use of standard kits. Fixing the catheter to the patient to prevent relative movement, in-line filters, and impregnated surfaces are called for in some cases.

Hospital-acquired infections put the patient at serious risk and extend lengths of stay.

Pittsburgh Regional Health Initiative

Pittsburgh Regional Health Initiative (PRHI), a supporting organization of the Jewish Healthcare Foundation, is a voluntary association of large and small hospitals, including VA hospitals; large insurance carriers; a large number of clinics and professional groups; and civic leaders covering western Pennsylvania. PRHI was organized in 1997 with the purpose of sharing information and improving the quality of care up to the highest level. Healthcare employs about 12 percent of the workers in the region and has $7.2 billion in annual billings. The region has a long and fruitful history of involvement in civic betterment by industry leaders and philanthropic organizations. PRHI took up the matter of central line–associated bloodstream infections.

METHOD

First, PRHI's partner hospitals observed the existing situation, pooling their information. This became the baseline against which further improvement would be measured. The partner hospitals agreed to update their information at least quarterly so that progress could be tracked. The CDC and other interested parties, including Highmark Blue Cross Blue Shield of Pittsburgh, joined in the project.

Upon reviewing the state of the art, the parties agreed that the existing CDC standard was the best available guidance. The hospitals reminded nurses and others of the importance of following the guidelines and confirmed supply quantities and disposition of supplies. No breakthrough in method, technology, or equipment was identified. Rather, diligent application of the existing guideline was urged. Observation followed by standardization.

RESULTS

The goal is zero infections. There is no specification short of that goal, and the intent of the program is to continue until the goal is met or at least approached as closely as possible. Figure 16.1 shows the progress as reported in the July–August 2005 edition of the PRHI newsletter. (The newsletter is free; sign up at PRHI's website: www.prhi.org.) The figure shows that the infection rate fell from 123 to about 36 infections per 1,000 patient-days of central-venous catheterization. That's good. More to go, but good so far.

Note that the chart shows all infections in one dot. No distinction is made between Hospital A and Hospital B. While each hospital has access to all the data and can make its own competitive charts if they want to, the fundamental idea of lumping everybody together in one chart has merit. All hospitals are following the same

Figure 16.1. Central Line Infection Rate

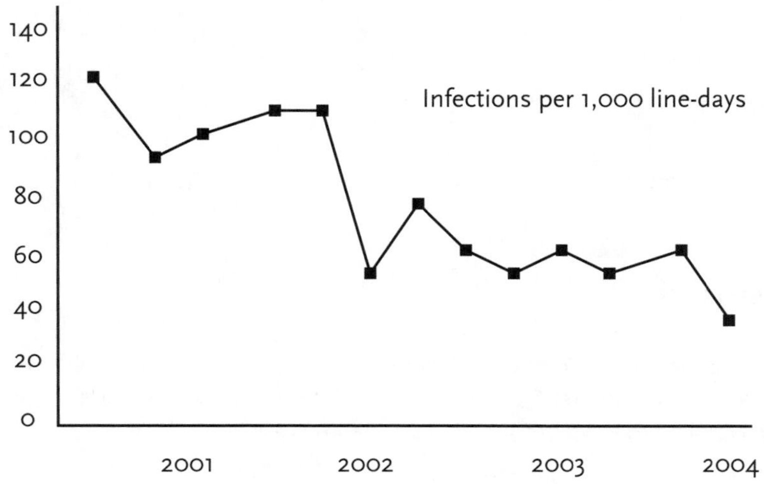

Source: Data used with permission from Pittsburgh Regional Health Initiative. 2005. Executive Summary Newsletter, July–August issue.

procedures, and the best group learning comes about from the biggest aggregation of experience. If a breakthrough comes along in the form of a new catheter coating, a new line filter, or a new cuff, that's great. Meanwhile, diligence is to be applied.

Public reporting of the progress is a good idea. PRHI's newsletter has been making periodic reports on this program. Tracking charts are a good senior management tool, allowing the progress report to be viewed at a glance.

FURTHER INFORMATION ON HOSPITAL-ACQUIRED ILLNESS

See the Appendix for information about the statewide (every hospital, every patient, every discharge record archived) report now available in Pennsylvania. This appears to be the largest reservoir of information on hospital-acquired infections and mortality, covering a very large population. The state's intent is to identify best practices so that others can adopt them. A worthy goal.

Note

Management at PRHI provided additional information in this chapter.

Reference

Centers for Disease Control and Prevention (CDC). 2002. "Guidelines for the Prevention of Intravascular Catheter-Related Infections." [Online article; retrieved 9/12/06.] www.cdc.gov/ncidod/dhqp/gl_intravascular.html.

CHAPTER 17

Discharge

Proactive discharge management is required to overcome local optima and free up bottleneck capacity for new patients.

BACKGROUND

Discharge management is more difficult than admissions management. Admissions management is, at base, reactive. The patient is right there, clamoring for attention. There is no corresponding self-actualizing clamor for discharge, and things, if left to themselves, will tend to slip. Freeing up a bed requires asserted effort by the discharge managers.

Discharge management needs to be proactive. Somebody needs to pay attention, make sure all the formalities are lined up, make sure the orders are written properly, and make sure that the bed is made up for the next patient—all in a timely manner. A hospital with 100 beds discharges 20 to 35 patients on a routine day. A hospital with 200 beds, twice as many. That's a lot of beds to make. As patient flow improves, the number of discharges per day goes up. More discharge work to be done each day. Every patient has special circumstances, so each case is different. As patient flow improves, the size of the discharge planning department is likely to grow.

Failure to provide a sufficient staff of discharge managers will be a barrier to patient flow—a self-imposed limit on patient flow.

PREADMISSION DISCHARGE PLANNING

With hospital stays down around three or four days, the discharge for the average patient needs to be done before the patient is admitted, or at least a good start on the discharge plan needs to be in hand.

In our admissions discussion in Chapter 12, we encourage giving preadmission sessions to teach the patient what to expect, to take care of paperwork, and to clear away any additional issues. Part of the preadmission session should be given over to discharge planning. Deal with these questions with the patient:

1. Who is going to drive you home?
2. How is your driver to be notified?
3. Can your driver come during the work day?
4. If you stay an extra day, can your driver adjust?
5. What size car does your driver have?
6. Who is going to help you when you get home?
7. If you're going to be on your own at home, who is going to look in on you?
8. Who is going to pick up your medication for you?
9. If you do not go home but rather to a care facility, what arrangements have you made? Do you have insurance coverage for a care facility? How will you get there?
10. What insurance coverage do you have for this hospitalization? Do you have insurance cards and identification cards?

These are routine questions, and the point here is that they should be raised and answered beforehand, not when the patient is lying in a hospital bed. The answers need to be captured and used as the basis for the discharge plan. For patients not getting a preadmission session, these questions need to be posed to the patient as soon after admission as is practicable so that some time is available to deal with special needs.

POSTADMISSION DISCHARGE PREPARATION

The admission order is the basis for estimating the discharge day, using prior comparable cases as a yardstick. Reconfirm with the responsible charge nurse periodically. Figure out how and where to find the doctor to get the discharge order written. Verify driver availability and communications. Line up any specialists, such as physical therapists, who will be involved in the discharge process. Line up housekeeping to remake the bed and room for next use.

For a hospital of any size at all, a good number of discharges will happen each day. Planning for one patient melds into planning for this number of patients. So housekeeping planning, for example, needs to involve housekeeping management to be sure that an adequate number of housekeeping teams are available for each coming day to match the projected discharge count. A standard time budget to make up a room should be set and actual completion times tracked to be sure that adequate staffing and supplies are being provided. A crisp notification method needs to be organized, using cell phones or pagers, so that a "patient out" list is updated constantly and the "bed ready" list is updated, too.

Following are some everyday issues that arise.

Hide a Bed

No, not that brand of sofas that convert to beds. This is "hide a bed" as practiced in many a hospital. A bed becomes available for a new patient, but somehow that information doesn't quite get communicated. It's a particular form of local optimization, and it interferes with patient flow.

If it is left to the local charge nurse to declare a patient to be out of the room and to notify housekeeping and then the beds-available control center, then lots of things can happen to introduce delay.

The fundamental one is that bringing the next patient into the unit brings a substantial amount of work for the charge nurse, who must interview the patient, determine a care plan, scare up any special bed equipment, and get the patient safely into bed and properly instructed. If the shift is nearly over, it is tempting to let matters slide until the next shift comes on. Or, the charge nurse can be quite busy taking care of urgent needs of other patients. Or, the charge nurse may not feel empowered to expedite housekeeping if no one appears to make up the room in a timely manner. Or something else.

Better to have the discharge planner take responsibility to stand in the room, wave goodbye to the outgoing patient and family, call housekeeping, log the call time, and call the bed-control center to forecast a bed in Unit XYZ to be available in N minutes. Then come back in a few minutes to make sure housekeeping got on the task.

Find the Doctor

Lots of doctors now use laptop and handheld computers to issue orders. This is to be encouraged. It's also necessary that the doctor not only "send" but also "receive," because the discharge order may need to be modified. It is not to be expected that doctors will take hospital interests into consideration; it is, however, to be expected that doctors will respond to reasonable requests from the hospital once those requests are made known to the doctor. Discharge orders are negotiated.

Find the Specialist

Physical therapists and other specialists may be involved in the discharge process, perhaps determining whether the patient is strong enough to go home or needs to go to a care facility. Determining which specialties are to be involved and scheduling the specialists are important to getting control of the discharge process.

The Checklist

All processes should be executed from a checklist. Processes, such as discharge planning, that include several disparate elements done at different times and probably in different orders, running over several shifts, should certainly be done from a checklist. Particular thought needs to be given to the meaning of the checklist when the circumstances of the patient change. If the patient stays an extra day, all the transportation boxes previously checked need to be unchecked and done again. Or if the family member calls in to say that the planned transportation is not going to be available at the target hour, more unchecking is to be done.

Attending to the validity of the checklist is a responsibility to be assigned to a specific discharge planner and not shared, because while the checklist itself is the most mechanical of things, keeping it valid takes concentrated thought. That means individual responsibility.

Keeping the checklist on the computer system is convenient. But computer systems are not known for the quality of their thinking, so the responsible discharge manager still has to do the thinking.

NEGOTIATED DISCHARGE ORDER

Let's look at the unfettered discharge flow in Figure 17.1.

Figure 17.1. Basic Discharge Order

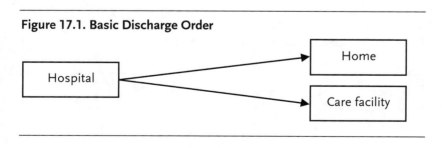

The doctor issues a discharge order, shown by the one-directional arrow, and the patient goes home or to a care facility. That's simple enough. However, this simple flow does not address any interests that the hospital may have. It is better to insert the hospital into this flow so that the hospital can get things right in the first go-around rather than chase things later.

In Figure 17.2, the bidirectional arrow means that there is a negotiation between the doctor and the discharge planner. The doctor holds the upper hand, so this is not an even negotiation. Even so, the hospital has interests that the doctor may not anticipate, and so there is necessary negotiation to be done. Better to recognize it, and do it every time.

For example, a patient comes in three times a week for radiation therapy. The same patient comes in with pneumonia, which is treated and that allows the patient to be ready for discharge in the afternoon. The doctor, thinking of the patient's convenience, may prepare the discharge order to say "discharge after Thursday radiation treatment." That may be convenient for the patient, and it may even be compassionate, but it is not consistent with payer rules. It is in the hospital's interest that the doctor write the discharge order to free up the bed today. If the patient comes again tomorrow, so be it.

Perhaps the hospital will decide that the compassionate thing is to let the patient stay overnight. Perhaps not. The point here is that that decision should be up to the hospital, not the doctor. The hospital will bear the burden of this compassion, not the doctor.

Doctors have the remarkable right under law to spend hospital money. The hospital has the collateral right to defend itself

Figure 17.2. Discharge Order with Flow Control

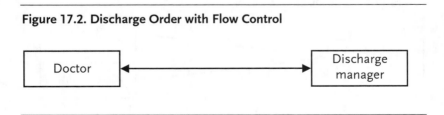

Going Lean: Busting Barriers to Patient Flow

by persuading the doctor to take an enlightened course of action.

DISCHARGE HEDGING

To hedge is to act in anticipation of uncertainty. Whether the patient is strong enough to go home or needs to go to a care facility is a decision that may be made on the last day in the hospital. If a care facility is ordered, a care facility needs to be found in short order, otherwise the patient stays in the hospital bed. If care-facility beds are almost always available immediately, then no problem arises. If care-facility beds are not always available, then there are at least two courses of action that merit consideration.

Playing the Odds

If historical data show that the odds of needing a care-facility bed are 62 percent for each hip replacement surgery, say, then the hospital can take options on that many care-facility beds each day, even if it has to pay something for the option. This course of action is amenable to modeling (forecast game playing), negotiation, and trial and error. Freeing up the bed makes room for the next patient and improves patient flow.

Buffering

To buffer is to decouple actions in time. The patient can be moved to a buffer facility for a brief period of time until a regular care-facility bed becomes available (see Figure 17.3). Some hospitals operate licensed care facilities for this buffering purpose.[1] This is a separate license. Admission to this buffer care

Figure 17.3. Buffered Discharge Flowchart

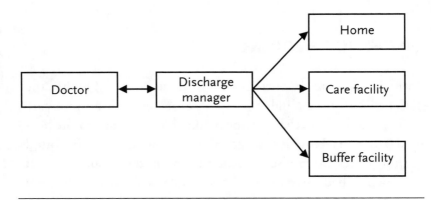

facility is distinct from admission to the hospital. This is a separate revenue event.

Because the buffer care facility is intended as a short-stay facility, patients transfer to a standard care facility as soon as a bed there opens up. (Keeping the patient in the buffer facility longer than the least possible time defeats the whole buffer purpose.) It is within a hospital's power to get a care-facility license, to set up such a facility, and to staff it. Having a buffer clears a barrier to patient flow. Not having one constitutes a barrier to patient flow. Recall that a barrier is a self-imposed impediment to patient flow. Not having a buffer care facility is self-imposed.

Paying the Patient to Go Home

Any hospital can wind up with financial responsibility for a patient who no longer needs inpatient care. The hospital may be faced with the choice of keeping the patient or paying for other medically appropriate care at some other facility.

Some postdischarge patients need intravenous antibiotics for four or six weeks but no other care. Medicare won't pay for home health, which leaves it up to the hospital. Paying a qualified home-infusion service provider to take care of this frees up a bed. Some self-pay patients are found to meet the qualification requirements for Medicaid coverage, but they are not yet enrolled with Medicaid. Getting enrolled can take several days. Nursing homes are naturally reluctant to accept the patient until the Medicaid formalities are completed. The hospital can keep the patient or guarantee payment to the nursing home.

Establishing standing contracts with home health providers and nursing homes to cover these situations generally facilitates rapid action for each patient when the situation arises.

EVER-CHANGING REGULATIONS

In July 2007, new Medicare regulations require that each acute care patient give an informed consent to be discharged. The regulations allow for appeal and review, a process that may take three days or more. If every patient refused to consent to being discharged, it would nearly double the average length of stay and thwart many years of improvement in facility utilization. How this is all going to play out is not known at this writing.

All regulations are well intended, and many arise out of specific instances that do require some rectification. Striking the right balance is challenging for all the parties involved.

Note

1. For example, Sharon Regional Health System in Sharon, Pennsylvania. See www.sharonregional.com.

CHAPTER 18

The Cash Cycle

While most payments can be looked up on a list, emergency department payments and some others are made by category. These are subject to statistical audit.

BACKGROUND

Emergency services, wound center services, and some others vary greatly in complexity, supplies consumed, and time required. Providers bill for such service by first assigning each case to one of five or six complexity categories and then by billing at an agreed rate per category. The provider is free to establish its own rules for assigning cases to categories.

The payer, then, has only to pay per category and to confirm from time to time that the provider is using sensible internal rules for assigning cases to categories. The payer will likely test the provider's traffic against comparable providers in the state or region. This is a statistical test. If the test raises flags, then individual records can be dug into.

We encourage management to track activities of all sorts. Tracking the bases for reimbursement is a worthy thing to do. The difficulty is that most managers don't know how to track six-dimensional values. Who would?

SELF-TESTING

Most reasonable people find multivariate statistics to be baffling. To overcome this barrier, we provide the following simple, but utterly sound, analysis. Consider Figure 18.1, which shows the distribution of cases for "This hospital" and for "Peer hospitals." The question is, are these two distributions about the same, or are they not? If they are not, perhaps additional management attention is required before the auditors get interested.

Here's how to proceed to make this understandable and easy to track. We reduce the hexanomials to one simple figure of merit. In this case, there are six categories. Tabulate the data in two columns on a

Figure 18.1. Emergency Department Case Mix

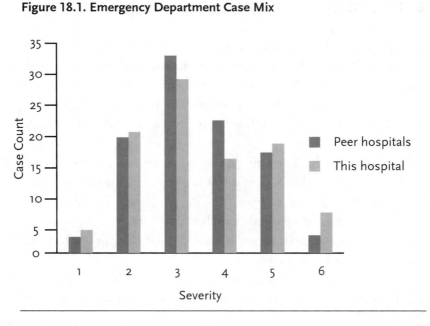

Going Lean: Busting Barriers to Patient Flow

computer spreadsheet. Tell your spreadsheet application, such as Microsoft Excel, to apply its χ^2 (chi-square) test. The response will be a percentage. If the response is near 100 percent, then the local numbers are "close enough" to the peer group. If the response is near 0 percent, then the local numbers are not close enough to the peer group. The cutoff value for close enough is open to argument. But, the number of things to argue about is reduced to this one number.

The two distributions in Figure 18.1 look quite a bit alike. They are both high in the same categories and low in the same categories. So, a glance at the graphs would say they might be close enough. Oops. The calculated value is only 31 percent. That means the likelihood that these two distributions are the same is only about 31 percent. That's probably not going to be persuasive to an auditor. Management attention, before the auditor comes in the door, might be in order.

There may well be perfectly valid reasons for the differences. Management, in observing the traffic mix, can use this simple tool to make the observing easy.

COOPERATIVE SUCCESS

The cash cycle includes payer and provider. While they share a community of interest in patients and care, their priorities are not exactly aligned. Integrating process improvement projects necessarily means reaching an accommodation on what to do first, who does what, and how to measure progress. Following is the story of one successful and ongoing project joining a major payer and a major hospital group.

Working together, a very large payer and a very large provider improve the cash cycle.

THE OUTCOME

- Accounts receivable aged more than 30 days, cut 43 percent
- Denials by provider reduced by 75 percent
- Denials by payer reduced by 95 percent
- Denial processing time reduced by 70 percent
- Cost per inquiry reduced by 52 percent

With more to come!

THE PROGRAM

It's no surprise that getting a major improvement in the cash cycle involves both the payer and the provider. What may be a surprise is that two giants[1] got together, not to point fingers at each other but to work together side by side to make the process work better for both parties.

Headquartered in Pittsburgh, Highmark, Inc., an independent licensee at the Blue Cross and Blue Shield Association, ranks among the nation's leading health insurers and is the largest health insurance company in Pennsylvania based on membership. University of Pittsburgh Medical Center (UPMC), based in Pittsburgh, is a huge healthcare provider, including 20 hospitals, primary care facilities, professional practices, imaging services, tertiary care, research, and pharmacies. UPMC is a world leader in organ transplants and a wide range of medical research.

UPMC has about 4,000 beds, supports medical centers around the world, and is the largest employer in western Pennsylvania with more than 35,000 employees. These are two very big operations, each with national standing. They have one key thing of common interest—payment of insurance claims. Both are appliers of sophisticated computer systems.

The two companies came together in 2002 and signed a ten-year service contract, including a joint commitment to fund $20 million in initiatives over the life of the contract. With common interest and this source of funding, the remaining question was how to move forward. To facilitate the launch, the two engaged Capgemini,[2] a worldwide consulting company. Capgemini was expected to phase out over time, as the two parties learned from their own experience and could do things on their own. Having a third-party facilitator is often a good idea. No matter how well intentioned everyone is, the facts on the ground are that there are always different interests, different ways of viewing things, different priorities, and lots of history. That's not just the case between companies; it's often the case between departments and groups within any organization. The third party can be an outside specialist, as in this case. Or, it can be an employee who has been trained in the art and who has no ax to grind in any particular case.

SENIOR MANAGER SPONSORSHIP

Tom Tabor is the CIO (chief information officer) for Highmark. Dan Drawbaugh is the CIO for UPMC. Both sponsored the overall program, conducted joint meetings, assigned senior managers to sponsor particular projects,

Information Week named UPMC's Dan Drawbaugh CIO of the Year in 2006, not just for healthcare but for all industries.

and maintained senior management focus on the joint program. While senior management sponsorship is important in any process improvement program, it is all the more important in such a joint program so that the teams can see a balance both in effort and support.

BIG PICTURE, LITTLE PICTURE

Aided by the facilitator, senior management, middle management, and professionals in joint meetings made rather long lists of possible projects. Some of these could be done quickly, some would take years, and some would require the next generation of technology. Note that the candidate projects were not corrections of known errors. Error fix-up was being done routinely by each organization. The purpose of the new program was to go beyond, to deal with issues that were not well understood, and to build into the future. Because no one was quite sure how this was going to work, they jointly decided to look at specific measures to rank candidate projects.

The two groups settled on ROI (return on investment) and TTC (time to complete the project). ROI has a direct meaning here, given that they were talking about money and its value in time. Faster payment, better ROI. Lower effort to get there, better ROI. TTC is always iffy in software projects, but the need here was only to rank projects in terms of taking more time or less than others. The same quality of time estimating applied to estimating all candidate projects.

The upshot is that applying these two measures gave the quite-reasonable conclusion that the two groups should start with projects with high ROI that appeared to be doable in a short time. That's a mathematical way of saying, "Go for the low-hanging fruit. Then, work your way up the tree."

DATA DRIVEN

How do two groups figure out why some claims get stuck in the system? Observation.

The assigned teams met around a conference table, looked at a claim, looked at another claim, looked at a third claim, and on and on. They decided that the only way to figure out how to improve the process was to get a solid baseline. Take a case, walk it through. Where did it get stuck? Take the next one.

Rather than jump in with a specific fix for each specific case, the teams were patient enough to build up a baseline of experience in which they could see patterns. Then, they looked to see what systematic changes could be made to fix a whole class of problems at once. That's hard work if you're doing it by yourself. If you're doing it with two teams—one of which has acquired patterns of thinking much like your own and the other of which has a completely different view of the world—then that's really hard work.

One meritorious feature of this joint process improvement program was that the solution was going to be right there in that room. They were not going to be able to assign the action items to somebody else. It was their issue, their solution to create, and their solution to make work.

DATA DICTIONARIES

One thing that the teams found was that they lacked a common understanding of the meaning of each data item to be entered into each other's computer applications. That took a lot of talking and even more listening. Eventually, some changes in documentation were made to accommodate the language, or perhaps the jargon, of the other party.

This is a common data-processing difficulty, exaggerated when two separate organizations are involved. It's also a common difficulty when two sets of accountants or two sets of engineers are seeking common terms. The added complexity with computer systems is that the computer doesn't have the common sense to ask when something doesn't seem to be quite right.

SHORT TERM, LONG TERM

At this writing, the two companies are about halfway through their ten-year commitment. Short-term benefits, as listed at the top of this chapter, are in the bank. Longer-term projects are continuing. One medium-term project has been to create a common dashboard to show operational status of the claims process, as in Figure 18.2. The data to be portrayed were selected by both teams.

It's called a common dashboard because observers in either organization will see the same dashboard and the same real-time

Figure 18.2. Claims Status Dashboard

Highmark–UPMC Unit Claims Status

In Process	
45 days	357
30 days	1,204
< 30 days	27,993

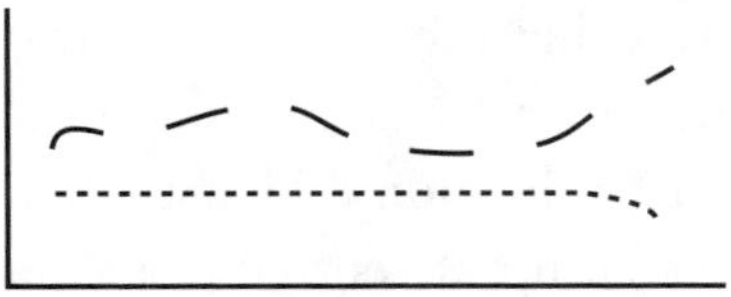

Finalized	
Item	Value
Count	9,714
Gross Amt.	$20,000,000
Denied Amt.	–$7,500,000
Adjustments	+ $ 50,000
Net Amount	$12,550,000

(Conceptual Portrayal)

Source: Sample used with permission from Highmark, Inc. and UPMC, Pittsburgh, Pennsylvania.

status data. That's a good way to reinforce trust—showing the same data. Nothing hidden under the rug, nothing up the sleeve. Just a neutral report on where things stand. Figure 18.2 is a simple black-and-white conceptual portrayal of the dashboard idea. The actual dashboard screen is in color and has hyperlinks to allow the user to drill down into deeper layers of information with a click here and a click there. The dashboard is not just for the computer operators. It's for senior managers, middle managers, professionals, and anybody who has a keen interest in the flow of cash.

EXTENSION

Highmark deals with many care providers. UPMC deals with many payers. It is in the interest of each to extend the benefits of these joint development projects to cover all those other parties. One can imagine a dashboard of dashboards so that senior management can tell what's going on at a glance.

FURTHER INFORMATION

A longer article on this project is available online at www. hctproject.com (search "Highmark") and in a publication by Montgomery Research (2004). The longer article pays particular attention to the macro-scale issues that arise in managing many projects in parallel over a prolonged period of time. Not many organizations can cope with doing more than a few projects at a time, so prudence is the watchword.

Notes

1. Management at Highmark and UPMC provided additional information in this chapter.

2. Capgemini's U.S. healthcare practice was acquired in 2005 by Accenture.

Reference

Montgomery Research, Inc. 2004. "A Success Story." In *Health Care Technology: Enabling Collaboration Between Payers and Providers*, Volume 2. San Francisco: Montgomery Research, Inc.

CHAPTER 19

Long-Term-Care Facilities

Residents of long-term-care facilities are vulnerable and require special attention to keep them out of acute care facilities.

BACKGROUND

It may seem that including the long-term-care facility resident population in a book on patient flow is a bit odd, given that these residents don't intend to go anywhere. Yet, these same residents constitute a disproportionately large fraction of the patient flow to acute care hospitals, and surely they are better off if their trips to the hospital are the minimum number necessary and are well executed in every case. Keeping these residents healthy helps in that regard.

IDENTIFICATION

Many residents of a long-term-care facility are not competent to identify themselves; at the same time, many of these residents resist wearing name badges and wristbands. Because these residents are long term, the permanent staff of the facility will get to know each resident by sight. But there are other nonpermanent staff who deal with these residents.

One volunteer—a retired registered nurse—told us that she goes to her community's long-term-care facility at lunchtime to help feed the elderly female residents. She sits at a small table with three or four residents and feeds them all at the same time, one after the other, spoon by spoon. Usually, one or two of her residents are on a special diet and are to be fed specific foods. That's fine, provided that this volunteer can tell who is who. Name badges are often not present, and self-identification is iffy. The residents tend to dress alike and fix their hair in the same style. The nurse-volunteer and the residence administration came to a workable solution by issuing photo-ID cards, not to the residents but to the volunteer. The administration first got written authorization from each resident, or family, to use photos for this purpose.

Long-term-care facility residents are taken by van to cancer centers and other outpatient services where identification is apt to be important. They are taken by van to acute care hospitals. Who provides the identification when the patient is delivered? The van driver? An identification system, something beyond name badges and wristbands, common between the residence facilities and the care-provider facilities, is certainly in order. If the same identification system can be extended to cover patients who reside in their own homes or with family, so much the better.

INFECTION

According to the Centers for Disease Control and Prevention (2007),

> Methicillin-resistant *Staphylococcus Aureus* (MRSA) is a type of bacteria that is resistant to certain antibiotics. These antibiotics include methicillin and other more common antibiotics such as

oxacillin, penicillin and amoxicillin. Staph infections, including MRSA, occur most frequently among persons in hospitals and healthcare facilities (such as nursing homes and dialysis centers) who have weakened immune systems.

Perhaps, each year, half of those who die from healthcare-acquired infection contracted MRSA and its associated effects (Karlowsky et al. 2003).

Residents of long-term-care facilities are of particular concern because they move back and forth between their residence and acute care facilities. They are apt to be infected, and they are apt to be carriers. They are also apt to be in communication with others, who in turn become infected. That carryover is more apt to happen at the residence than in the hospital, so the residence's administration has a special interest in knowing who's infected and who is not. Residence workers can also become "colonized," which is of even greater concern. Colonized persons can spread the infection even while exhibiting no symptoms. Workers are not apt to be the ones to bring MRSA into the residence, but they can acquire it from one patient and spread it to others.

During a five-day period in 2005, all 250 long-term residents at the Veterans Administration (VA) campus in Pittsburgh were screened for MRSA. Thirty-nine patients were found, quite unexpectedly, to be colonized (PRHI 2005). All were asymptomatic. These patients were separated from the general population and provided treatment. The high colonization rate—about 16 percent—convinced VA-Pittsburgh management that 100 percent screening of new residents and periodic rescreening of all residents were necessary. Special screening equipment was acquired to make this practicable. VA management also redoubled its efforts to encourage good practice among healthcare providers, including wearing gloves and gowns, sterilizing instruments, and lots of washing of hands.

VA-Pittsburgh had a breakthrough—a negative one—when the high MRSA-colonization incidence was found. This called for a compensatory breakthrough—a positive one—namely, the new screening procedure and new policy. This pair of breakthroughs brought the facility up to the level the administration had thought, innocently but wrongly, to have achieved beforehand.

PREVENTIVE CARE

Preventive care for residents of long-term-care facilities is important for their continued well-being. One consideration for this population is prevention of pressure ulcers/bedsores. The standard preventive method is to change soiled diapers promptly and, separately, to turn the resident in bed during the night so that the resident is not in the same position for long periods of time, with the resident's weight bearing on particular points. Wet diapers are less of a concern given the absorbent capacity of adult diapers these days. Detecting when a diaper is soiled is not impossible, but so far the known solutions are uneconomic. Turning patients in their beds has a known solution—namely, telling the orderlies to turn the patients. That's only part of the solution; the other part is making sure that this gets done.

Studies by Mark Friedman[1] (2007), president of AugmenTech, Inc., in Pittsburgh, show that patient-turning tends to be omitted from the tasks of residence workers and that worker-maintained manual records are unreliable. Why does patient-turning get omitted? The workforce undergoes high turnover because the pay is low and the work is heavy. The high turnover means that the caregivers, especially on the night shift, do not develop any affinity with the residents. While the work schedule allows enough time for patient-turning, upsets to the work schedule are frequent, with workers called away from their scheduled tasks to deal with some urgent matter. Whether or not a resident got turned cannot be known by observing the resident in bed. And so, when the shift is over, the invisible tasks get omitted. Worker-maintained task checkoff lists are unreliable. What to do?

Various technical solutions are known but not widely used. Assigning the work to pairs of workers would cost little or nothing, and the task checkoff lists might be more reliable. Better yet, before doing anything, observe.

Observe the flow, not of the patient but of the workers during a shift. Make a diagram of the worker's movements. A simple sketch is enough. These are called spaghetti diagrams; see Chapter 8 for examples. These diagrams need not be done for every single worker, just for representative workers over a few shifts. Management will surely expect to find that the worker starts out with the right materials on the cart, moves from room to room in the simplest way, and wastes no motion. Reality may be that way. Or, reality may not be that way at all.

How many trips to supply points? How many return trips to rooms? How many out-of-sequence room visits? How many diversions for more urgent matters? The answers can be most informative. Such a study may well reveal that requirements have changed since the work was originally laid out, necessitating extra trips, and that things just need to be reorganized. It may reveal that requirements have grown to the extent that even with reorganization, not enough time is available to do all the tasks 100 percent of the time. It may reveal that the compensation system needs to be adjusted to make sure that sufficient diligence is applied to patient-turning.

Notes

1. Mark Friedman holds a Ph.D. and is a licensed nurse's aide, giving him special qualifications for researching long-term-care facility operations.

2. Management at the VA provided additional information in this chapter.

References

Centers for Disease Control and Prevention. 2007. "Healthcare-Associated MRSA." [Online article; retrieved 5/28/07.] www.cdc.gov/ncidod/dhqp/ar_mrsa.html.

Friedman, M. 2007. Personal communication with the authors, January.

Karlowsky, J. A., C. Thronsberry, M. E. Jones, A. T. Evangelista, I. A. Critchlet, and D. F. Sahm. 2003. "Factors Associated with Relative Rates of Antimicrobial Resistance Among Streptococcus Pneumoniae in the United States: Results from the TRUST Surveillance Program, 1998–2002." *Clinical Infectious Disease* 36: 963–70.

Pittsburgh Regional Health Initiative (PRHI). 2005. [Online newsletter, September; retrieved 9/12/06.] www.prhi.org.

Recommendations Summary

Here are specific things that can help patient flow and that only senior management can do.

1. Create a patient-flow control desk to centralize admission control.
2. Create a discharge control desk, which may be the same as, or colocated with, the patient-flow control desk.
3. Create an observation unit distinct from inpatient units.
4. Create a licensed, buffer care facility.
5. Encourage the use of hospitalists as attending physicians.
6. Redesign all compensation systems to favor patient flow.
7. Urge all senior managers to spend time observing.
8. Encourage standardization.
9. Sponsor a small number of breakthrough projects.
10. Require progress-tracking charts on everything of interest.
11. Encourage caregivers to ask, why is this patient still here?
12. Count length of stay in hours, not days.

Hospital-Acquired Infections Reporting: A Beginning

Hospital-acquired infections harm patients, slow down patient flow, and give healthcare a black eye. A Pennsylvania program is beginning to provide solid data.

THE 2005 PENNSYLVANIA HOSPITAL-ACQUIRED INFECTIONS REPORT

For some years, Pennsylvania has had a policy of providing hospital-by-hospital information to Pennsylvanians so that informed choices can be made by healthcare consumers. This policy now includes an annual hospital-by-hospital report on hospital-acquired infections. The first report, issued in November 2006, deals with data for calendar year 2005.

While there have been many prior reports on the incidence of nosocomial infection, this is perhaps the first large-scale report done in such breadth and detail. Pennsylvania has a population of about 12.4 million, and it has large cities and small towns, major medical research centers, and small community hospitals. Pennsylvania demographics are skewed somewhat toward the elderly. Therefore, this report is reasonably representative of the nation as a whole, with the study covering about 4 percent of the national population. As demographic studies go, this is a very large sample, lending credence to the results.

The sponsoring organization is the Pennsylvania Health Care Cost Containment Council—PHC4 for short. The report, "Hospital-Acquired Infections in Pennsylvania," and related information are available on the PHC4 website at www.phc4.org.

To have apples and apples for meaningful comparison, the hospitals were all instructed to use the definition by the Centers for Disease Control and Prevention: "an infection is a localized or systemic condition that (1) results from adverse reaction to the presence of an infectious agent(s) or its toxin(s) and (2) was not present or incubating at the time of admission to the hospital." Data were contributed by 168 acute care hospitals. Cases involving children under the age of two and cases involving transplants and burn patients were excluded. Data were taken from regular patient records. Three hospitals with "special electronic tracking systems" all showed higher incidence rates. Because that anomaly was unexplained at this writing, those hospitals are excluded here, although the report contains those data in a special category. This exclusion leaves 165 hospitals, ranging from very large to quite small.

Table A.1 captures statewide data at a glance; this table is directly from the report. As seen in the table, infection brings an increase in mortality from 2.3 percent to 12.9 percent. Taking these numbers and scaling up to estimate the national numbers gives about 62,000 excess deaths and about $90 billion in excess cost due to these infections, nationally. Daunting as these numbers are, they appear to be below previous estimates. Infection brings an increase in length of stay, from 4.5 days to 20.6 days. A bed occupied by a patient with infection is a bed that cannot be used by another patient, so infection brings a reduction in useful inpatient capacity and is therefore a barrier to patient flow.

The original idea for these reports was to provide a baseline against which each hospital's future performance can be measured.

Table A.1. Statewide Summary Data

	Number of Cases	Infection Rate per 1,000 Cases	Mortality		Average Length of Stay (in Days)	Average Charge
			Number	Percent		
Statewide	**1,569,164**	**NA**	**38,716**	**2.5**	**4.7**	**$33,267**
Cases with infections	19,154	12.2	2,478	12.9	20.6	$185,260
Urinary tract	11,265	7.2	983	8.7	16.8	$123,725
Surgical site	1,615	5.2	68	4.2	14.5	$132,110
Pneumonia	1,824	1.2	452	24.8	24.3	$256,133
Bloodstream	2,602	1.7	540	20.8	27.3	$282,276
Multiple	1,848	1.2	435	23.5	36.0	$400,262
Cases without infections	1,550,010	n/a	36,238	2.3	4.5	$31,389

Source: Used with permission from Pennsylvania Health Care Cost Containment Council.

Figure A.1. Infections Versus Cases

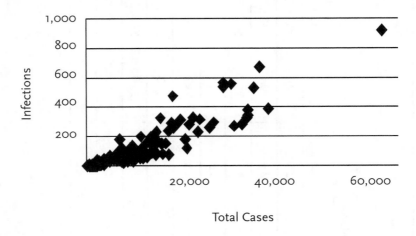

Total Cases

Source: Used with permission from Pennsylvania Health Care Cost Containment Council.

Let's see what this report tells us on the basis of just one year. Figure A.1 is a plot of the number of infections versus the number of cases. If everything were exactly the same at all hospitals, a straight line would result.

This plot shows that the number of infections increases as the number of cases increases. Indeed, seven hospitals report no infections at all. These were at the small end of the scale, but such success is to be recognized wherever it is attained.

At any one case count—say, 25,000 cases—there is a spread between the highest and the lowest infection counts. That may mean that some hospitals in that size range are doing better and have something to say to others that are not doing so well. Perhaps so, and that surely was the point of the study in the first place. However, it is tempting to see more in such a cloud of data than is really there for us to see. Figure A.2 is a plot of the same data in the form of a histogram of infection incidence rates (the number of infections divided by the number of cases for each hospital). Just look at the shape of the histogram, which shows how many hospitals fall into each segment.

Figure A.2. Acquired Infections Occurrence

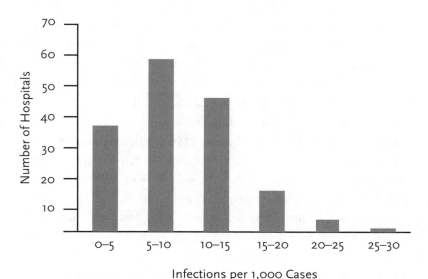

Infections per 1,000 Cases

Source: Used with permission from Pennsylvania Health Care Cost Containment Council.

The horizontal axis represents the infection rate (infections per thousand cases per year). The vertical axis represents the number of hospitals having that infection rate. Per the figure, about 60 hospitals fall in the 5–10 infections-per-thousand-cases-per-year range, and about 3 hospitals are in the 20–25 infections-per-thousand-cases-per-year range. There is no new information here; this is merely a rearrangement of the same data shown in Figure A.1.

Again, look at the shape of Figure A.2. This looks like the Poisson distribution from any statistics textbook. The Poisson distribution is the distribution of discrete events that happen with low likelihood for a large population. Poisson governs the number of people who are standing in line in front of you at the supermarket checkout and the number of customers who go to the bank on Thursday during the lunch hour. Poisson governs the number of emergency cases that turn up on a Saturday night when the moon is full.

Before the Pennsylvania study even started, any analyst would have said that if all hospitals follow the same practices to preclude infections, then the results will follow the Poisson distribution. Because the results (Figure A.2) do have that Poisson look, all that can be said, so far, is that the data do not show any subset of hospitals to be doing better than any other subset. The first year's outcome cannot be distinguished from random fluctuation.

To the extent that the fluctuation is random, hospitals with a good score in 2005 may get a bad score in 2006, and vice versa. The only way to know if some hospitals know something special or are doing something different from the others is to see who gets better-than-average scores over a time period of three, four, or five years. The likelihood that any one hospital will find itself below the median infection rate for three years running by chance alone is one chance in eight. For hospitals above the median, the same. So, hospitals that show good, or bad, results for three years running are worth some study because they are doing better, or worse, than random fluctuation would make likely. On the other hand, a hospital that is above the median one year, below the next year, and then above again the following year is showing us nothing at all.

This report is a good beginning. The next annual report and the one after that will merit very close scrutiny.

About the Authors and Contributors

Amy C. Smith is director of case management/utilization management at Western Reserve Care System in Youngstown, Ohio. Mrs. Smith is board certified in both advanced practice nursing and nursing administration, with expertise in project management, case management, and performance improvement. She is a certified Six Sigma Black Belt and holds a master's degree in medical/surgical nursing from Gannon University and a bachelor's degree in nursing from the University of Pittsburgh. This is Mrs. Smith's third book on hospital management.

Robert Barry, Ph.D., author and consultant, has more than 40 years of experience in corporate management, specializing in trustworthy systems. Mr. Barry holds a Ph.D. in engineering from the University of Pittsburgh, is a graduate of the Harvard Business School, holds the rank of Master Black Belt in Six Sigma, is an adjunct professor at the University of Pittsburgh, and is special consultant to the board of the International Christian University and Hospital in Kinshasa, the Congo. Mr. Barry holds 11 U.S. patents. This is his sixth book on hospital management.

Clifford E. Brubaker, Ph.D., is professor and dean of the School of Health and Rehabilitation Sciences at the University of Pittsburgh. He holds additional professorial appointments at the University of Pittsburgh in rehabilitation science, neurological surgery, and the McGowan Institute for Regenerative Medicine. He holds adjunct appointments in the Robotics Institute, School of Computer Science at Carnegie Mellon University, and in the School of Life Science and Technology at Xi'an Jiaotong University in Xi'an, China. Dr. Brubaker has contributed to research, education, and service in the fields of biomechanics, rehabilitation engineering, and assistive technology for more than 30 years. He received his bachelor's and master's degrees from Ball State University and his doctorate degree from the University of Oregon. Dr. Brubaker is a past president and Fellow of the Rehabilitation Engineering Society of North America, a Founding Fellow of the American Institute on Medical and Biological Engineering, and an inaugural Fellow of the Biomedical Engineering Society.

ABOUT THE CONTRIBUTORS

Mark Hernandez serves as senior managed care/access to care specialist within the Army Medical Department (AMEDD) One Staff TRICARE division of the U.S. Army Medical Command. In this position, he provides expertise for strategic planning, organizing, staffing, decision support, and policy development. He also serves as a health systems program specialist and supervisor, overseeing the operations and policy formulation of AMEDD programs in the areas of managed care, access to care, and regulatory requirements.

Becky Southern, R.N., M.S.N., has 25 years of professional and management experience in pediatric trauma nursing, home health administration, and women's and children's service line management and as chief nursing officer for a 400-bed community hospital. Ms. Southern is a member of the American Organization of Nurse Executives, a member of nursing and nurse administration honorary societies, and a board member for the Caridad Center. Ms. Southern is a Six Sigma Black Belt.

Mark Viau, RT(C), CRA, FAHRA, has 28 years of professional and management experience in radiology, imaging services, surgical services, cardiology services, respiratory services, anesthesia, inpatient transportation, and central scheduling. Mr. Viau is a past president of the American Hospital Radiology Association (AHRA) and a Fellow of the AHRA. Mr. Viau is a Six Sigma Black Belt.